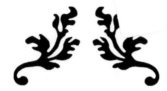

SOUL CODES

Remembering your Mission

ZOE ANA BELL
Sydney, Australia

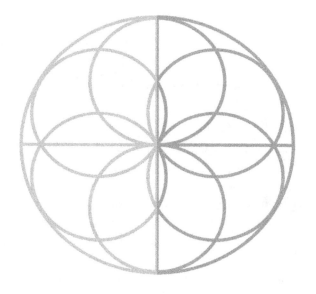

Soul Codes – Remembering your Mission- Zoe Anna Bell
Book 3 of the trilogy series: FREE WILDFLOWER CODES
Publication 2nd February, 2022 RAW Publishing
ISBN: 978-0-6481776-6-1

DEDICATION

This is dedicated to all seeking deeper meaning to life, the crazy ones that know they are here to do great things and are part of *The Great Healing Mission for Humanity.* The ones that wish to tap into the magnetic sensually deliciousness of life and break away from 3rd Dimensional physical game of power, fear, corruption and control. The chosen ones that chose to come back to clear up the destruction and dance our way to restore the Earth. The misfits that never felt heard growing up with no one to understand their Souls depths. The ones that learnt to walk alone by learning how to heal themselves. The ones that never gave on finding the magical place inside no matter how much they were rejected.

To my children, Jake & Charlie, may this be a guiding light as you venture through life and remember the powerful co-creators that you are. You chose to come back, perhaps as activators, illuminators, Warriors & Wizards of Pure Source creation to shine the creative expression of You. This is your life and you each have a divine purpose on Earth. My love for you is unconditional and eternal. Be willing and fearless to follow your heart, even when others reject you.

To my infinite Soul, what a wild crazy ride. Every day my eyes, heart and Spirit experiences a state I cannot describe through words, as it is beyond description. Angelic wings expanded with fearless width, embracing each layer of change and weathering each storm with moment-to-moment presence. It is going to a rocky road for many as the chaos crumbles the old structures, beliefs and what many are holding onto in self-perpetuated misery.

Even though I do not know what is beyond, I have an inner sensing of what is coming, and it is magical beyond words or what the human mind can currently comprehend. It is good to be home, here on Planet Love.

To my Soul family, each day, the energy of love ignites as we re-uniting with our multi-dimensional abilities awakening. Each strand of DNA and Code weaved into the magical tapestry of life all are playing a key role. As Children of God, future beings we are here to dance and play with one foot here grounded on Earth and the other in the Spiritual realm.

As above, so below, as within, so without and a sacred place where heaven meets Earth. This is not for those that are looking for science to prove anything as resonance is felt and the darkness of the void all to be explored. I am not here to convince you. I am here to evoke the love within you and stir the insatiable creative explosion within You.

To my teachers, past, present and to come, infinite students of life and all who have impacted my life in unique ways. To lovers, guides, fellow weavers and mirrors, you are each your own inner Guru.

To the reader, enjoy the finale of the *Free Wildflower Codes*. What a journey this has been to bring this into a digestible and relatable offering. May this be the compass to assist your continued navigation to knowing thy Self and the Universe.

Pillars to build upon the foundations presented from the previous two books with the intention to *Awaken and Activate Your Soul Mission* into knowing who you really are and to be in service within the new Earth.

I invite your child like innocence to place everything you know on pause and to enter this book with a mind that is yet to know. This is the best way to learn, grow and evolve beyond the known and from the blank slate.

Tabala Rassa meaning to clear the slate.

Have fun implementing what resonates, in all-ways. Take it or leave it, it's all an invitation to become curious to explore deeper into the depths of You and we are accelerating at a rapid rate.

Enjoy Soul lovers,

Let us begin,

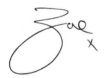

CONTENTS

FOUR WORDS

UNAPLOLOGETIC

COMPASSIONATE

COURGAEOUS

SPIRIT

INTRODUCTION

It is time to de-mystify what is tripping you up and introduce Key Principles to support to re-wire both the body and the mind and shift from duality into Unity. Each key component crafted to awaken your human potential and I encourage you to fearlessly follow your intuitive heartfelt desires, which requires checking in with yourself, as much will be stirred to be brought to the surface. Be fearless warriors that choose to walk in peace, the Feminine Rising is here, and it is time to shine!

More often than not, each of You will have experienced a path perfectly aligned to shape who you are now and who you are becoming beyond the story, that you are holding onto. Perhaps, a past of overcoming adversities, limitations, pain and inner suffering and for many seeking the way to be free. As you discover the shadows in your closet and what you don't want others to see or know about you, you have a choice to be brave, accepting who you are being in each moment and through conscious awareness of your reactions and with diligent action you begin to reveal your gifts. By doing this you play an active role in healing humanity, as you are beginning with Self. The healing process works from the inside out and is best described as a re-birthing and death cycle that happens as many times over is required. A dying before you die to the habits, behaviours and resistance that is blocking the view. This is a path of initiation to polish your unique Soul by design and activate your purpose with the gifts to share in your creative expression.

Within these pages are Codes within codes and some being hidden within others, all intricate pieces of the clever puzzle, a journey of discovery through self-realisation. A puzzle that fits together as you integrate codes, and the signs will present within your living environment of the day-to-day as a part of your growth. Yes, the entire Cosmos is within You as you are the Youniverse and We are all part of the multiverse, that is the ONE.

My intention is to bring insight, provoke curiosity, restore clarity and awaken your inner confidence so you too begin to live life on your own terms. I am here to share tools to explore and sharpen for your next expansion and integration of them into your life. There is no beginning or end, as when one journey ends another is beginning, and codes are constantly activating and upgrading. The key is to be present yet relaxed, poised yet excited to face your fears, to greet each challenge as it is here to strengthen your trust and faith in God (Self) and to walk into the unknown. The Universal Law of Free Will symbol on the book cover will magnify what is within your life, be it fear or love. Life on Earth is a training ground and no matter where you are currently at is divine for you and what is about to unravel as a spiral and even chaos is vital to navigate. This book gives you the tools and I am simply a bridge to share what I know and there is so much that I do not yet know.

The density of the suppressed past story is heavy, take a moment to pause and enquire within. '*What am I holding onto?*

To grow and leap you have to be willing to be teachable and face challenges of Soul initiation. There is no pass go free card or avoiding doing the inner work and no one is coming to save you. This book will not do it for you, it will provide ways to keep you on track and nothing happens without daily and consistent action.

INTRODUCTION

Within your body matrix there are cells, and within these cells strands of DNA with codes that switch on gifts and your Superhuman powers. Each codon is assisting the collective frequency of consciousness to evolve. This translates to the greater the density that you transmute (inner work) then you greater your capacity to embody light. Leading to a bodysuit that can emit higher states of consciousness (Love) to guide others home.

Are you ready to play a key role in raising the free-Queen-see on Earth?

There are forces working for and against your alignment, and that are all here for your growth. Some mask as the light, as 'False light.' I will refer to them as 'Moths', as they often play both sides of the light and the dark. The Galactic adventurer has the ability to explore polarities to distinguish the lie/illusion fed since a child and see the truth, that it is all of it. These are aspects of initiation as a result of choices made as only then can you truly understand good from evil. Life is a game and even making the so-called wrong turn will open up a karmic thread to then find your way back to the clear path of the *'Middle way.'* The light or dark are within you all as they co-exist, and the balancing of the scales is a key aspect to the path. I mention this with discernment as when you open up the higher chakras, then you become open to everything. It is key to know the distinctions and to know when you are being *The Cosmic Slut*. Open to everything with an energy field that is getting fed off by external forces and drawn into spells and remember the Power of Choice and Free Will.

The false light and evil forces feed off you and IT wants to keep you stuck in limitation, distracted by illusions, hooked in the forces of sexual manipulation, corporate conglomerations, indoctrinated beliefs and the ultimate poison, separation of our species! Even separation plays a role to

3

activate the path within and the games being played is so intricate and masterful it would take a lifetime of study to inner stand it. It is a distraction and is not why we are here!

The demonic forces at play will tempt you with power and a thirst for control! That has a road ends in self-destruct, the end of the line. Welcome to the 3rd Dimensional physical game and the inverted Matrix many are living in. Where there is peace there is corruption and this is not about this or that as that would be separation and duality. You have a choice, wallow in self-pity, keep complaining or evolve. The key is to restore inner balance beyond inner reaction, awaken fluidity of equilibrium and to know thy Self. The dance of flexibility and neutrality and to Master the game you are IN. To see that you have played a role in everything you reject and deny, as within an awakened state of peace, love, respect and harmony there is no separation, only what IS. The path of serving God is towards the right and a path to restoring natures ancient inner knowing.

The truth is love.

Love is consciousness

Unconditional love with no boundaries,

Fear is unconsciousness

Fear separates humanity

INTRODUCTION

Self-love is to be mastered by each soul

To step away from the HIVE socialised mind

Until then, honour Your boundaries!

Yes, a no bullshit badass!

Be ruthless to avow.

Since releasing my first book in 2017 there have been huge upgrades and thinking shifts and much not knowing as I continued to explore. I have been slammed back to what felt like the beginning, on my ass until the next message of relief presented. Getting slammed is like being caught in the middle of a huge set of waves pinned under until I stopped fighting against the flow and to surrender into the trusting of allowing. To be in a state of presence with nowhere to go except be in that moment. I no longer say RESET as this term has been misused by the global elitists to create spells of confusion in this Spiritual war. It is time to simplify life, be diligent to what you feed and remember what really matters.

Many are stuck in complaining and miss the point of everything is playing out to assist free will, personal freedom, and liberty to evolve beyond the 3rd Dimensional physical Matrix. To heal the 3rd density is to shift beyond the body, transmute fear, dissolve resistance and be brave to make the changes. This is the leap in consciousness happening right now where the individual is stepping up with the courage to be disliked, addressing their shadows and into the heart of compassion and forgiveness. This is 3rd to 4th Density. The heart is the sacred doorway into higher states of consciousness and the level of the soul of 5th density. The gateway to Heaven on Earth and the love frequency. Your mission is to continue upgrading the physical vessel so that when the sonic waves of higher Free-queen-see hits the grid the physical bodysuit goes with us, and all multi-dimensionalities come online. We are each playing different roles and no density is better than the other.

The cosmic intensity has been naturally rising impacting the life force energy in all to assist to prepare the leap. From late 2018, I went from high vibe excitable to exhausted flat in my back, naturally upgrading in dreamtime/sleep. Countless times commanded to lay down by Extra-terrestrial beings to rest, trust and allow. My body-vessel worked on by Arcturus light-beings, Pleiadeans, Lyra beings and other ET Brothers and Sisters. I've observed being suspended within bright green and aqua sparkly goo which was a higher dimensional healing substance of love and peace. Each event that took place I'd be out cold for 44 minutes in a deep sleep. Post the upgrade my eyes would take 2-hours to recalibrate and now in 2021 when it happens the turnaround is 11 mins or so. Post the upgrading event I would walk around looking half stoned, peaceful, slightly euphoric and giggly like a child that was just given *'Space dust'* candy.

I shared on podcasts and interviews my experiences and realized that others were also having very similar experiences with light beings / ETs. In Jan 2020, Angelic beings guided me to shift my daily practices into sacred rituals of freestyle play all to accelerate Soul remembrance as a Pleiadian to assist activation of the crystalline quantum grid, all of which I integrate each day.

It was around the same time that I had moments where the only thing I can call it was *'free-falling into the unknown, the void.'* This was during breathing practices of holding my breath and once passed the 5-minutes mark without breathing it was as if time collapsed. The next time I looked at the clock 11 minutes 11 seconds has passed! Holy F*ck and I have experimented with this many times. During the holding I feel deeply relaxed with no desire to breath and a thought....

'It must be time to breathe.'

How can the unknown and a space of nothingness be described? It cannot, as it has to be experienced, beyond labels, description or being a thing. I am sharing an experience and it was deep relaxation, like being home, the unchangeable Oneness. Like you, I am an explorer within the experiences presented.

Some breathing practices I timed for fun and curiosity and the angels would communicate with numbers and specific sequences. This is key to not take life too seriously, and when you feel the righteousness attaching with opinion, observe it and let it go.

Do you see double, triple digits or number sequences? Are the angels looking to communicate with You and are you present to listen?

As mentioned in *Breaking Free* each of You have an original blueprint all to be activated and carved out as your divine Soul/Life path. When synchronicities increase it is a signal of rapid upgrading and being on the most aligned path. Teachers present into your conscious field all in divine timing and many are in unexpected disguises. Perhaps a lesson to be faced or rejected as once the lesson is done, it is done. If a lesson keeps happening, you are missing the root cause or perhaps you are playing a role for the other. Life may require stepping away in silence and it can happen super-fast. Remember this is your own life so be present enough to stop getting drawn into another's drama or karmic merry go-round as it is not your dharma or path.

The journey of the heart is raw and messy all to ease and rip your heart into growth and expansion. Each direct interaction is profound with meetings all supported by the angelic realm, perhaps psychic healers, mirrors and friends within your circle that trigger the fuck out of You. Be grateful for these lessons, to see clearer in your soul remembrance.

You have an entourage of angelic beings that walk alongside you. They are always listening, ready to support and guide you on this journey. Remember that You are never alone. Be willing to listen as when they speak it is felt and requires all your attention. The Scribes assist me with my writings.

Humanity is calling out for fearless leaders of Self to assist in Healing Humanity. The rebellious ones have been finding one another like lighthouses beaming brightly and here we are, it is now all happening. If you are reading this then this is calling You and I am aware that this has been on the backburning for a few years and this mission of awakening humanity upon the ascension path.

As I continue to grow and evolve it has become apparent to document and pass insights, teachings and integrated wisdom on. As like You, I too shall leave this physical plane of existence, I am simply playing a role in this body as an infinite being. As You begin to see beyond the veil of the illusion you are being fed, it will become initially noisy wondering what and who to believe and trust. People's fears often play out to protect their inner pain and to attempt to make you wrong. Wondering if you've joined a cult and passing judgement. People you love, yes, your friends and family may reject your ideas as they see life differently to you. Being rejected is part of the greater plan. I now Ask God (higher Self) and the entourage of Angels around me to guide to where I am needed to serve, as a Child of God.

Avoid a lifetime of struggle and stop attempting to convince others that you are right, and they are wrong.

Do you and be you and choose to walk the path of your inner truth. Each lesson requires having a healthy self-esteem to remind you that no matter what is thrown at you, said behind your back, or disapproved of you always return to Self.

We the Rainbow Light Warriors that have your back as we came here to do the dirty work deep in the darkest shadows. We the Guardians of Light and the Galactic Alliance are here to guide you home by walking our talk.

See all with gentleness as what other's think of you is none of your business, they are a mirror of your old self, and it is time for loving kindness, compassion and remembrance. It is also not your place to judge as what you most reject you are yet to love within. Acceptance is key as you and I are all in this together.

There is no one place better or higher than the other as this is entitlement and arrogance in motion. Stay true to what feels good, know right from wrong and do right that bring no harm to others with the knowledge you have at your fingertips at the time of your conscious choices. Remember free will so nothing external impacts your inner presence of love, unless you choose to allow it to have power over You.

Stay the F*K in your own lane.

Nature is your home, a playground to play, explore, seeks solace and receive guidance from Spirit. The elementals of the sunlight, moonlight, stars, wind, water, fire, clouds are you Brothers and Sisters, as are The Trees Nation, Mineral-stone Nation and Animal people Nation. Respect the whole harmony of life as Your Soul family and 3rd dimensional birth family all play a vital part in your ascension. The path of ascension is the path of Mercy, to see the divinity in all. 2021, is the year of Redemption and will continue into 2022.

Nourish your mind, body and spirit to allow your inner wisdom to birth and reveal your fearless heart. Being banished you from the circle or tribe is integral to your evolving path as a path of initiation. Address your inner vibe and release what has outgrown the upgraded frequency. There is beauty in seeking solace alone to honour inner healing and when Souls are meant to be in your life they will loop back in perhaps years down the track. If your path goes against the grain of what you have been led to believe, then you have a choice.

Nothing I suggest is to force or convince you, it is all an invitation to question everything, even your own opinion, and be the explorer of self.

My advice, be relentless in self-responsibility of your daily inner practices as these are the souls medicine to reveal heart clarity. Once your passion and purpose lights up online it can no longer be ignored as there is no going back to the so called 'normal'. Whatever the fuck that is?

Never banish YOU to keep others comfortable as your divine Soul mission requires zero outward confirmation or validation from others. When souls turn their backs on you, even family members, they are turning their backs on the aspects that are yet to learn to love and possibly accept in Self. Be the Mirror of light and radiate love.

Learning is infinite and humanity is yearning for healing.

Every one of You holds the answers in your sacred DNA, that is if your DNA is still intact from not being seduced by the fear agenda of the so-called plan-demic.

Each day is a transition of ascension to seek knowledge, mercy and apply it through integration and to be diligent in all your choices. To know what is morally right or wrong and good or evil and to honour free will. Free will is not about going out and doing anything you wish to. Free will is a feeling within and acting from a place of respect, peace and beauty for all. The Grandfathers of Spirit ask everyone to know what is in your sacred heart, to find and feel that which is the centre of life. The Sun rises in your own heart that is the guiding father and the

Rising of the waters of the mother and the re-birthing of innocence as the Child of God.

Life is many shades of grey and everything all-in-between. Look for other rare individuals that are a splash of bright colour upon the canvas of life. Perhaps you are one of those rare individuals that dares to explore beyond the lines of conditioning and social obedience. Look out for these are they dare to shine in the world of many shades of grey as guiding lighthouses.

You each have a story. I am not you and you are not me, meaning all lessons and experiences have their own colouring direct for you. Once You transcend beyond the false Self (identity, ego and labels) you recognise the higher Self, Source and God. The I am Soul, and We are Soul. And within the we are soul we each bring a unique tonality to bring into Universal and Cosmic harmony.

The way You see the world will differ, depending upon life lessons, insights gained, or not. The home you grew up in with your parents or caregivers' religious beliefs and their family values all influence the colouring or smudging of your canvas. The painting of Your life.

As You reach your teenager years, a pivotal time of stepping into adulthood and the *rebellious Self* you will have seen the bigger picture playing out. This may have been brainwashed out of you by school, fear of stepping out of line and your well-meaning parents that also forgot about their inner power of questioning systems, rules and orders. This is the time you began to form your own beliefs and values now influenced by friends, pop culture and social media. This is where a sense of belonging to a tribe outside the family home begins. A need to belong, a place to fit in, to been seen, respected and heard. A human desire to feel loved.

The challenge is, many now in adulthood are stuck in the painting, thinking and believing that is their life. Many forget that they are the painter and not the painting and no matter the painting and scene, you can change it whenever you choose. You are the Artist and the Author of your life.

Be the change!

Step up, take self-responsibility, badass ownership for actions and accountability for all choices. It is a moment to moment step up!

Many are living for experiences and are missing the wisdom to be unveiled within the lessons. Some are lazy with integration, and some give up before they get to reap the rewards of inner freedom and to be liberated from the story.

Many have been seduced by tyranny and fear and have given up freedom. They have also shortened their lives. It will all play out; the Universe is constantly balancing.

The fact you have this trilogy in your hands is a sign that there is something that has intuitively guided you. A gut feeling with a magnetic pull to explore the unknown and see what unfolds, this is known as a strong intuitive message. Every written word is infused with activation codes, raw passion all to align exactly for You. A message from my heart, spirit and soul and it is Pure Love.

There is no destination as fluidity does not travel in a linear way. Yes, goal posts will shift so see this is a kaleidoscope adventure. Anything that makes you feel uncomfortable is evoking an emotion to be acknowledged. This is a key to your own healing. Have goals with a willingness for flexibility of change as this will assist in resilience, adaptability and growth. All keys to flourishing into an evolving Earth, a place where heaven meets Earth, and this is within you.

The mind plays games of judgement and fear of what others think and this is one of the greatest enemies in your life. Only you can choose for you. The path will have stones along the way, some to step over, others around and others may be thrown at you! Be ready to be nimble like a ninja to leap, duck and weave. Take solace, retreat into nature, attend to the inner work and see life as the playing field of warrior initiation to nourish your growth. From next level of awareness, to the next level, and so forth. It's like space invaders and your spaceship vessel needs your attention of love. It needs one commander and a support team, and it requires clear navigation all directed by a fearless heart that never gives up on the mission.

Waking up is never pretty, it is chaotic, messy and multilayered with deeply humbling moments. For many it was too much, and they made other choices within that lonely moment of the unknown. Yes, checking out with suicide. They may have only needed to hear the words:

'Are you okay, it is not your fault, and I am here to listen.'

The path of suicide as I understand it means the individual has an opportunity to come back to re-learn the lessons. The next time with greater contrast of pain, all to wake-up from their dreaming within the story of their own self-created nightmare. This is my own opinion, and if you have lost a loved one to suicide, I am deeply sorry for your loss and pain.

INTRODUCTION

Those who have gone too soon, I feel leave us a message, perhaps a red flag to wake up. I honour my unapologetic presence each and every moment, a reminder of the three beautiful souls in Breaking Free that died too young. They were each giving me a message to wake-up, of which I now understand.

I am sorry it took me so long.

If You continue to place blocks and walls around your heart, you become disconnected from those that love you and disconnected with your authentic spiritual essence. Those living in greed with excessive wealth and the high walls of protection of property to keep others out are perhaps wrestling with biggest inner demons of all. The media, news, magazines and large corporations will feed on your insecurities, doubt and fear. The ultimate illusion served up in the family home as tele-a vision, creating programs in the psyche of the young pliable mind of children.

This can keep you trapped, disempowered and is one of the ways for mind control. It is time to be wise up and be discerning in all your choices. Some movies have great codes to assist your DNA activation and others are there to activate fear. I watch a movie from the Observer perspective, fully aware and present. Trust your instinct beyond external influence of the matrix and question everything.

Life is about finding the keys that are unique to un-fu3k yourself.

You are the ultimate key holder to find your way back home.

The time is now to unleash the limitless and magnetic You. This is the beginning and goes way deeper than what I am in a position to write as much requires my presence in person. I am activated to get this out into the public, it is as simple as that.

The Mind-Body and Spirit Principles provide practices and rituals to implement into daily living. Each is there to assist you to feel connected upon a grounded stable base upon which you build a functional, flexible and powerful structure. A body-mind vessel that has the ability to hold the energies as they increase in waves and bandwidth of light frequency. The heavy carbon density of the past/trauma/programs to transmute into a crystalline light structure. With a powerful state of inner wellbeing, you create optimal states for restoring vitality, health and wellness to rise as the Seer and Truth Seeker.

Infused within this book is ancient wisdom related to your creative expression and to unlock mysteries in sensuality and intimate connection beyond lust. It is my pure intention to play a pivotal role in healing the rage and shame in the collective consciousness by guiding others how to heal trauma and restore sensuality to its innocence. I am one of the ground support team for the transition of Masculine to Feminine consciousness into Divine Union and guiding Sacred Sensuality.

Bit by bit, layer by layer, codes and insights will reveal. You will crack, melt and you will have to honour rest and space to allow each upgrade. Life may persuade the process through meltdown, break down, maladies, and even injury. Things like purging, screaming, sobbing, laughing, a mini rest will become a daily ritual of birthing your Source medicine. There is a pause of 'not knowing', in the in-between or nothingness and everything.

This suspension of free falling is a magical place to drop into once you let go of the knowing (having to know the outcome). You have to let go of what you think you know to allow the inner knowing of your intuition to reveal. There is no force, it is a path of allowing and facing your greatest fears and often what is holding you back, like the wounded heart when it comes to understanding unconditional love. You are showing up to play the infinite game.

You cannot know the unknown as the unknown is experienced and cannot be described as it is formless. It is in the pause of not knowing that many gave up and checked out with suicide, and many have attempts in this window. Have the courage to be patient within the pause, sleep is a great restorer for clarity of thought. Ask your Guardian Angels to surround you and hold you as you are truly never alone. You are beginning to trust. As You dissolve all that you think you are and shift beyond the body, senses and mind you experience or state than cannot be described, it is remembered as an unchangeable formless omnipotence.

Meet your fear, invite in trust and begin to have faith in being supported, and divinely guided by Source, a higher force that is omnipresent within this magical Cosmos and Earth. You get to play here, and you and I are all interconnected.

Trust and Faith are your wings, and they only develop by initiation of challenges.

There is no urgency, take as much time as you need as you get there when you get there as no one can live your destiny, as the Author of You.

You and I are all in this together.

Meet Tink, symbolising Freedom

The Rising of the Feminine.

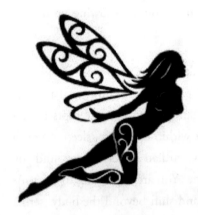

CHAPTER 1: BEING HUMAN

"We meet ourselves time and time again in a thousand disguises on the path of life". - Carl Jung

SOUL FAMILIES

As Star seeds becoming Star blossoms You chose to come back to assist clearing up the karmic debris and many of you have been born into adversity and experienced immense inner suffering. I am reminding you again that you chose this life and each experience activated something within to learn lessons and remember your Soul mission. What was remembered before coming back was forgotten at birth and this began the path of navigating life, the lessons required, and many times repeated till DNA was activated and gifts revealed.

You each have a Soul family and groups that go way beyond blood lineages, and it is a deep knowing that each are here to assist your evolution in consciousness.

No matter if you agree or not, this is my opinion and take on life. Life is a choice and the quality to which you live life is also a choice. Humans have become disconnected, focusing outwardly on short term rewards others rather than clearing up their own shit storm! It is time to honour and remember your natural human essence of love and to be humane is to demonstrate compassion, understanding, gentleness, and benevolence towards all beings.

Humans are often bitchy, judgmental, mean,
intolerant, and plain nasty as they have forgotten their
natural state of loving kindness and innocence.
Zoe Bell

Imagine, you are the centre of the Universe as life will deliver to you what is most requited to enable your expansion, the wanted and the unwanted. It is not what happens, it is the meaning you give it, and from there the empowered choices you make. Being human, is about having experiences, of both pleasure and pain. And learning to let go of it all, what you think you know, and to experience the depths within, alone and in silence. It is within the silence that you become closer to Self, as you are God.

You are made up of energy, a bundle of juicy flesh, that consists of billions of cells, communicating with one another 24/7 and an electrical matrix of electro-magnetic waves. Energy cannot die, it morphs and changes form. You are all part of the whole, and it is also time to remember your wholeness, the light- the dark, the yin- the yang, the sun-the moon, the day- the night. The shifting frames of contrast that you experience, and one can never exist without the other. It is your identification with what you believe is self, the Ego, that creates the biggest illusion of all. Your reality (experience) becomes an illusion of your original reflection, of what you think and belief to be true.

It is only when you can gain recognition of the illusion being an illusion, that it dissolves. Even free will is an illusion as life will deliver experiences to what is aligned for your Souls greatest expansion. You have to begin to see who you are not, and it is only then that the reality of who you are will arise out of the dark.

Most humans are thinking without awareness (non-awareness), and the compulsion to enhance one's own identity, with association with a place, person or identity. This is the structure of the Egotists mind. The sense of 'I', and all importance of an illusionary sense of the identity veil. The ego strives for identity, attachment, control, obsession, and a relentless un-quenched thirst for more. You are not your body, your pain, and you are not the suffering.

To let go of that aspect of the "I", is death itself.

You have to be willing to die before you die.

You must meet your own ugliness of judgement.

You must begin to trust and have faith in what is unknown.

It takes courage to continue to peel back the layers, to be seen, judged, naked and raw, and honour the dark inner shadows of shame, denial, lust, and guilt. Be willing to be rejected and abandoned again and again, to explore beyond, as the al-one.

All that can be known is.

I know that I am,

I exist

I am Soul.

We are Soul.

Make it your mission to keep exploring deeper, to look for the 'I', the one watching, talking, and to watch the one watching, as this has to be experienced and practiced. To do this every day until peace envelopes you. You are not your story, or the painting. You are the artist with the brush and life is about taking action beyond the flaky wishing upon a prayer and living in false hope.

PERFECT REFLECTIONS- 'SLUT SHAMING'

This has been a driving force of my journey, rising beyond shame. Shame is a disease of the collective and I am here to expose the truth. It is time to see the Mummy bloggers and the slut haters with love and compassion. You are all reflective mirrors, and to say you are not judging another again and again, is a sign that you are indeed judging when no one is listening and watching behind the scenes.

Let's dive into the psyche of the *'Mummy Bloggers and Slut Haters'* that huddle together for safety in their groups, bitching and complaining of the rightness and wrongness of the woman that embraces her sensuality and sexuality. They refer to this kind of women as a slut, whore, and a threat to what she embodies. This woman radiates her full goddess feminine Source essence and is unafraid to express it. They create public humiliation around this kind of woman, in an extremely nasty and passive aggressive way.

The Slut haters will do everything in their power to banish, maim and disown her. If this was their daughter, they would shame her for the way she dressed, the make-up she wore and the way she chooses to express her free and raw sensuality. Even worse, they would banish her from the family home and from all connection to her community. This would continue until she yielded to their rules to conform thus suppressing her free expression. Lured into false love and acceptance so she could feel worthy by them to receive their love. An invitation into their slut hating group with a sacred soul scarred, sucked dry and left for dead on the inside. The beginning of a socialised mind and many of these hide behind and within religion.

Can you see a similarity in the games played out by the government and social police of 'Karen's' reporting or threatening those that chose not to wear an obedience mask or get vaccinated for the C19? The public shamming, voices silenced and attempts to ostracised in a community? The low vibration of shame, blame and guilt all to manipulate the vulnerable, conditioned into control tactics and the below the line living. This is the fear that keeps you stuck in your own matrix known as a prison of the victim consciousness.

Be the one that dares to stand up and pursue your heart no matter what others think. The separation within society is a separation within the individual's inner psyche, and the more one shames, then the less one is able to love the aspects they've made wrong.

This is an opportunity to activate your personal free will and protective resonance of freedom by diving even deeper into the inner work on You. Earth is your planet and is calling your voice, your heart and the beating of your Soul drum.

Evolving consciousness of the human is an inside job and rejection is a step to shift beyond codependency of a group, family or tribe. There is always a silver lining of the Greater Plan. Groups are everywhere in society and it takes courage to look deep within. The groups that label others are motivated by two things.

- Fear
- Shame

"To these women, it is time to nourish what has been shamed and banished within. I have love in my heart for you, kindness, humility and forgiveness, as you didn't know any better. I feel your pain, as the shame and guilt run deep, and for many it is multiple generations. Until you begin to love the aspects that you have blamed, and forgive yourself, then it will continue. Now, you have this awareness, it is you that is judging and banishing your true sensual desires and needs, and I welcome you home, as you are loved'
Zoe Bell

This is a message for all the brothers and sisters who have felt shamed and banished by society for your variety of sensual and sexual choices, you are loved.

'I will not be banished or put you on the street, no matter what I will love you, and I will never banish myself again' Zoe Bell

Be clear in your boundaries and own it when you start placing ultimatums and restrictions as you fear of abandonment. The one who 'over-controls' is lacking in trust or self and the other. If you are with someone have the courage to be honest and when trust is broken, then the door gets covered up with armour and requires transparency. Some men and women seek affection, adoration and connection outside the relationship as they are hungry for intimate connection without a verbal stream of bitching and complaints.

As part of my soul remembrance was a phase working with female singles, and couples to evoke a deeper connection of mind, body, and sensual healing. For nine months I was an Intimacy Coach with a few select High-end clients and I chose who I worked with and when. This involved Soul intimacy, and firstly, building trust with the woman, was key. I was the glue to unifying each soul with self, and within intimate relating with one another. I was exploring the unknown and discovered that I was able to orchestrate three-energies into one pulse with ease and apparently this is a fine-art. This was remembrance of The Rose Lineage Teachings and codes of the Higher Priestess healings and Sacred Sensuality of the Pleiadean teachings. A path of initiation into activation of DNA remembrance and in the experience gain clarity to my path.

I was the woman living in fear and self-protect so I understand how women feel threatened by me and have had many women take from me with no respect of asking. A lesson as I had taken from women as I was living in fear, shame, competition and survival. I am here to assist heal the deep rage around sexual oppression, sexual trauma, sexual shame and feminine disempowerment. Everything you see playing out is an aspect within you to accept and breath more love into. Everything is choice. What are you consciously chosing?

The energy weaved is known as Prana. Prana is the Sanskrit word for life-force, which is Cosmic energy permeating the Universe on all levels.

As mentioned in *Wildflower* the life-force energy is sensual in-nature. I re-activated what had switched off by guiding men and women how to work with the Lingam (penis) and Yoni so that energy can shift out of the genitals and towards the heart centre and into higher states of consciousness and ecstatic bliss. I continue to share more wisdom on this topic to connect the sensual-life-force and abundant energy free of shame or guilt, as this is the healing Spirit, known as KA.

There was a large investment with this exchange of deep soul intimate connection. I created a service that bridged the gap bringing the sexual into the spiritual, so that was less drive to seek it outside and to heal the scars within their relationship. A path to unify and this deeper level of intimacy into intimate connection with open communication. Until one has walked the path of healing themselves and a path of life mastery by inner-standing sensual energy in the highest of regard, then to be of service to others may lead to the one giving feeling drained. I loved the experience as an aspect of gathering wisdom as it felt like the wisdom from lifetimes incarnated. I was exploring sacred initiations of the divine and I live life with no regrets, gratitude for each step.

I respect escorts as they are playing a role as we have all been there in this life or past lifetimes. I believe, many in the sex-industry are wounded at the root and sacral chakra's (1st and 2nd energy wheels) that requires inner healing. There is dilution of sacred energy, sexual manipulation and souls that are unconscious and unaware of what energy is. It is time to raise consciousness out of the genitals and into a higher frequency of Spiritually Holy and Sacred Sensual connection.

Raising consciousness is not about mindless fucking, it begins with self-ownership and responsibility for all choices and emotions. This requires honesty, respect and integrity. The faster you ascend, then the more you will communicate on a level beyond words, telepathy. Transparency is freedom of the lies. Valuing and respecting sensual energy during intimacy is vital as there is always an energetic transfer. The impact on an escort's yoni may take years of inner healing to clear, as I witnessed this in clients. DNA can remain within the body as stuck energy for up to seven-years and karmic shedding of unhealed trauma. This is sad, as the body is a temple, a sacred kingdom/Queendom and many women are seeking external validation and choosing this from a place of low self-esteem and low self-worth. This is relevant to all souls that have explored with many partners.

I am an advocate for openness, honesty and owing all your sensual desires. It is time to be shameless and to express the truest You. The truth is both men and women love to have sex and explore pleasure, and it is the shame and hiding with infidelity that are the demons. A healing space for deep transformation, and soul awakening safe boundaries was always established. The intention was healing and connecting with a soul on a deep, spiritual and intimate level. The process included releasing blocks, de-armouring the trauma-pain-body, and activating areas that were sleeping. The intention was to re-unite what had been misused, misunderstood and ready to be brought into purity and wholeness.

At the beginning of 2019, my energy shifted in frequency, and it was clear this was not the exact path. More clarity was to reveal as there was no need to touch intimately with my own vessel to evoke the healing. I began to explore activating others from a distance and explore where I no longer touched the individual. Always, place your energy first, and trust self through sensing. Honour the sacredness and have no shame with your journey, as it is all a path to refine.

Be brave to be real, raw to be vulnerable and always stand in your authentic truth. Risk being seen, judged and alienated as once you wake-up, there is no going back. To go back and do nothing is to suffocate your Spirit and Sacred Soul. Take as much time as you need and know that when you are being in your raw authentic truth of love, forgiveness and compassion in your heart, then others will begin to wake up and be inspire by your silent and relentless action.

HONOURING THE INNER MASCULINE

You were born into this world as sensual beings of vibrational substance and as a baby you had high peaks of surging testosterone and oxytocin. You and I explored the world through our senses. Touch, taste, smell, and sight. Life would have been a truly sensual experience, and this is a key to your evolution, as this was living in a state of orgasmic bliss. It is your humaneness that thrives for direct sensing experience.

No matter your gender you each have an inner masculine or an inner feminine. There will be within each of you an aspect you have shamed from being expressed, a thirst for sexual pleasure or perhaps, lustful fantasies of being devoured by multiple souls. The inner masculine is the primal desires expressed in raw sensuality, sexual freedom and desires to be physical. The aspect that desires to taste the rawness of both men and women, to pin him down and ravish him whole. To dance between dominance and surrender, fearless and courageous and to unleash her inner Source power.

Her spirit and flame were untamed and fierce, like a wild stallion.

The aspects you were told to tone down, like having too much drive, too much passion and determination are aspects of the inner masculine. The fighter that was told, girls don't fight, to sit down and allow the men to carry the load. The inner wild that is bursting to be free, that had more desire to run with the wolves and men than as they hunted their prey for the village. To run wild, get messy in the Earth, care not for looking pretty, roll in the dirt and unleash her inner roar! She was seen as untamed and dangerous, as her presence hurled men into lustful desires of no return. The women would throw stones at her, as they saw here as a distraction, a threat of their men. She was made to be the one wrong, and this is where the introduction of *'slut shaming'* began. It was the primal masculine that was being willed to learn how to control his lustful desires, restrain himself and each playing a role in consciousness. In saying this to become free is to let go of the resistance that you are holding on to and I am not talking mindless fucking and having no conscience to your actions. It is time to *re-wild your inner masculine and* forgive the hidden aspects you have shamed. It is time to see you are both forces within and to allow the shame to dissolve and witness the humour of it all.

This is for every woman, as you will not be able to see it until you explore your own darkness and embrace the aspects of you that love to get dirty and nasty. This begins a magical reveal of soul love and a welcoming of wholeness. Imagine the lioness awakening from a deep slumber and begin to hear her roar and purr shamelessly. The healing of humanity rests in the healing of the inner masculine wound is key in women. To let go of all control, unravel in wild surrender and allow the Sacred Masculine to be the container and protector he was created to be, as together they reach higher dimensions of cosmic bliss existence. It is a dance of the most magical weaving of energies. The Feminine Rising is not about women, it is all about the rising of the creative and magnetic forces with all as the path of ascension and evolving consciousness.

THE POWER OF BOUNDARIES

A very relevant code is to honour *intimacy boundaries.* For many there is a block around receiving love and a letting in love. It takes trust and a willingness to explore raw vulnerability in sensual pleasure. This is a magical journey to give yourself permission to *fully let go and moan'* and say exactly what you desire.

To command it by being direct!

Say no to what you don't want, and never be afraid of the power of your voice. Until you can own your no with confidence, the yes will be half-assed effort. Life will present many Nos in choices with relationship or sexual offers, and when you have fully got clear on your no, then yes' presents in abundance.

Many teenage girls are getting judged for saying yes, by peers, and parents. It is time for teenage girls to be able to make the same choices as teenage boys. If we look at maturity and emotional intelligence, a teenage girl matures emotionally faster than boys. This is also determined by the way sensuality is discussed within the family home and the attitude of the parent and caregivers. The power of yes, may be to explore with other girls, or boys with boys and this is perfectly healthy. It does not mean you are gay!

The teenage and young adult ages of healthy sensual exploration and learning about your body through sensations. As a nine-year old, I explored with other girls and then in my teenage years, 20's and I now proudly embrace my free choice of sensuality. This is purely an energetic connection, and what aroused me in moment-to-moment presence. This is about moving past the biological man and the biological women, as within our matrix there is both the masculine and feminine energetic forces.

Your natural state of being is love. Stop shaming your sisters or brothers and support their choices and free will and consequences of those choices.

It is powerful for all to own their yes. To combine sensuality with love is key where both fully open up their heart. Sensual pleasure intertwined and the breath whilst ravishing one another in the moment. Many women have a higher sex drive than men, and it is time to embrace your potent wildflower /pussy ladies. Others may judge your choices, call you names and all that BS, yet, as long as you are expressing your truth, then be that! Find a union to reach higher states of ecstatic bliss, that words cannot express, and it begin with self.

INNER REFLECTIONS

Read this through a couple of times, then close your eyes and follow as best as you can. Allow your guidance to guide you into your inner depths and be willing to trust and allow.

- Find a place where you can be still, quiet and uninterrupted.
- Gaze to the tip of your nose and softly close your eyes.
- Allow your eyes balls to relax deep into the eye sockets, like precious pearls on silk pillows. Allow the breath to be gentle (not forced) as you breathe in and out of both nostrils.
- Have the lips of the mouth lightly touching with the tip of the tongue lightly touching the roof of the mouth. A space just behind the front top teeth.
- Become aware of the gentle flow in and out of the breath and rest into this present moment.

- Stay here noticing the flow of breath in and out for as long as you like.
- Awareness with zero force, a process of allowing.
- When you feel guided to. Ask your *old self*

- (Name), ... what are you making wrong?
- (Name), ... what are you holding onto?
- (Name), ...what do you need right now?
- Allow space for the message to arise. Avoid looking for the answer as this is the wrong approach. It is all an invitation for the intuitive message of the higher self to come through beyond the mind (ego).

There is no right or wrong answer, as it is the ego (false self) that questions. With practice this becomes more refined and can be use in a moment-to-moment basis in all your personal and professional interactions. A technique to enquire into the higher-self and more of the way to communicate in full transparency.

The mind is noisy and to still the duality of the mind takes disciplined daily practice. Until one can transcended past the noise of the ego, the wise inner aspect of mind will be unheard. There are many ways to escape the bondage and the Vedic meditation was a way that worked for me and many I have passed it onto.

HEALING THE SEPARATION IN THE COLLECTIVE

Society is creating a greater separation of blocks and walls between people siding against one another. The hardest concrete walls to crack, as the ones within self. They are rigid, bound in arrogance, fear and entitlement as the cement binds them. The walls serve to protect the raw feelings and often hidden sensual desires, and many are living in a state of shame and numbness. They are ignorant to their own fears, and this is entrapment of the Soul and the collective *Victim Consciousness.*

Many women are afraid of their sensual power as they have been told its wrong and this thankfully, there is a shift, yet some are misusing their Source power by being disrespectful to men and this has to stop. There is a difference when a woman has embraced a healthy inner masculine, healed inner wounds, and owns her voice with gentle self-confidence. She lives with high self-worth and radiates pure love. An eternal inner flame that burns bright. She is inspiring and kind to all she meets as there is no external threat from anyone. This woman has embraced and learnt to love her shadows and radiates her gifts and superpowers to the world with grace.

There is a 'breed' of woman that landed powerful positions and has adopted a masculine exterior. She learnt that to get to the top, she must act like a man. She is mean to younger female team members as she feels threatened by their beauty and also the fear of them taking her position. This woman has some serious inner masculine wounds to begin to heal and honour as on the inside she is numb. There are *'men hating and penis hating'* women in power and this is where the feminist movement went off kilter. Feminism as a movement began with great intentions and lost its balance with a wonky, one sided view on the world, feminine patriarchy playing out.

I have witnessed women in full throttle of attack mode and the behaviour is ugly with unconscious groupies cheering her on. She is publicly putting men down, like a tit-for-tat, you put me down, so now I will do the same to you. I am all for equality in what each Soul contributes, and it is to be based on quality and contribution of unique gifts and nothing to do with gender fairness.

Men and women bring different things to the table, and this is where it gets messy. I will do my best to give points on all sides as really the only separation is in self.

I feel that feminine consciousness will see a shift as what I have learnt from womb healing is, there are times of a woman's menstrual cycle that are times for her to be in her own space. This internal process is rich in allowing creativity to be revealed and the wisdom that presents at the sacred time of her period. Women being shammed for having periods, talking about periods at work I feel is reason why the bitterness has increased and many becoming more conditioned like men.

The sacredness of surrendering and the power of allowing has been lost and this is shifting within the whole of society. 2020, created the perfect opportunity for connection with self, seclusion, stillness in nature and the 9-5 buzz placed on pause. This creates a wave of contrast were returning to work there was relaxation, introspection and contemplation instilled into more of the collective consciousness. Many women aligning with moon and their menstrual flow as they were less stressed and stepped away from the action based masculine environment. This consciousness shift of reconnecting to the feminine can shift the entire frequency of a room, thus assisting businesses to align more with the rhythms of nature and balancing of the polarities.

This is almost contradictory; I can hear the men.

Yes, I am sharing the possibility that during a woman's moon flow of the first 2-3 days she does not go to work or go to school and instead commits to deep womb work. This will be a vital key to balancing the evolving Earth of the Feminine Rising and supporting women for the passing on of the sacred wisdom. This is not using your moon flow as an excuse to play hooky or the manipulate others this is to be honoured as the grid lines activate the lei lines to support the leap into the 4th dimensional shift in consciousness.

Equality is an inside job, in all ways.

WOMEN WANTING SPECIAL RULES OR EXCLUSION FROM EVENTS?

If women want equal rights, then why are they asking for special ways to travel safely? I see it from all sides. Understand this, if you are walking around in fear afraid of being attacked, then you are inviting in that exact resonance! The pink carriage that was implemented onto trains for *women only* in 2019, in Australia I see as bait to the sexual predator. I am calling out the obvious as this is being pushed by the Neo-feminists and penis hating men!

Some women treat men in a disrespectful manner which is verging on abuse and many resorting to bribery which is threatening and illegal behaviour. There is media coverage about workplace harassment against men, yet many of the men are also getting the hard deal of the basket. I see this as a problem of the collective and when this happens, one has to always rewind back to see what wounds within self. Wounds that are raw and are not getting the loving attention they are crying out for. Men stand up, owning his voice and in his power and many women are squealing abuse, yet they are the ones that are the predator in disguise.

This is for every Soul, beyond biology. Address your inner wounds by owning the role you played to attract the situation, do the inner work and stop shaming others!

SOCIAL TOXICITY OF THE INNOCENT

Sadly, many teenagers are distracted by social media of sexy selfies, porn and this is a very different ritual to ancient times. They think is the normal and many young girls and young women are basing their inner worth on how many likes they get on Instagram and Tik-Tok. I have witnessed the bullshit playing out and when it comes to being 'street smart', many teens are less convoluted that the adults. Mind manipulation begins early and much that is driven in pop-culture is demonic with a satanic agenda.

The pink elephant in the room is Human Trafficking which is modern-day slavery and involves the use of force, fraud or coercion to obtain some form of labor or commercial sex act. 'If under the age of 18, force fraud or coercion does not need to be present.'

600,000-800,000 people are trafficked across international borders every year.

80% are female and half of them are children. U.S State department.

2 million children mostly girls are sexually exploited in the multibillion-dollar commercial sex industry - Information from Operation Underground Railroad

You place any picture onto the web, and it is straight into the dark web and this I've had to accept in my lack of awareness from pictures I shared openly.

There is separation in the collective with those that are speaking up to save the children and those that are choosing to remain in ig-norance and blinded by the plan-demic. You can turn this around and guide your children so that their innocence and safety is protected, and their freedom and human rights are honoured. Sadly, more are burying their heads in the sand to the human trafficking industry than courageously speaking up. Many are so invested in the internet they are ignoring their inner child and family that wish to play and connect in nature. If you ignore it then you are a part of it, period! You and I are here to Save the Children and reclaim the innocence within. Many adults hide in shame, blame and guilt with lustful desires and there are many fucked up people with wacko tastes!! Right now, year 12 children are being herded like cattle here in Sydney for mass jabbing of the 'so called solution to this plan-demic.' We will witness mass genocide, infertility and as a parent it is horrific to witness so many unable to critical think or see the bigger picture of the A-gender, those that have been jabbed are no longer fully human.

To begin to shift, be willing to open up conversations to learn from your teenagers as their DNA is more advanced and probably more intact than yours.

- Awareness begins with loving kindness, compassion for each individual to see what they are feeding and innocence being over-sexualised.
- The inner work is simple once you get a taste of the sacred medicine.
- Know when to shut the fuck up and always listen to your child.

- Never question or ignore a child's VOICE
- Be brave to address your inner shadows and sexual trauma
- Begin to heal your inner child
- Sit down and learn to meet and be with self and all your ugliness.
- It is magical when the layers of old shame melt away and forgiveness of self and honour sovereignty.
- Be a guide to support your children and teenagers into the rights of passage into adulthood by learning to explore the wilderness and take responsibility for your life.

- Be ready to open up your homes and arms to children that are the victims of the greatest crimes of humanity, as global healing will be required.

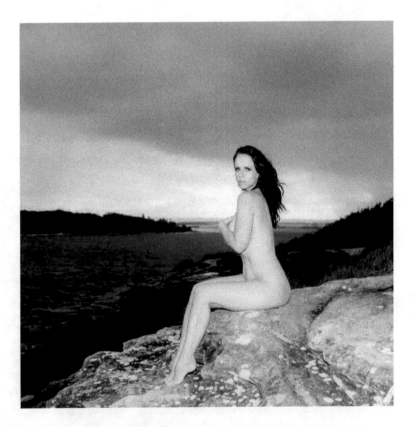

Taken from RAW- a Key to a Woman's Heart & Soul

This is the embodiment of a sensually awakened woman that celebrates her raw and wild Spirit. I am at home in nature, and it is time to restore innocence into what has been misused, abused and over-sexualised by demonic forces. This picture is not porn and not posted either for sexual gratification, let us together raise the bar. This was being free in my skin and a part of my own sensual evolution beyond the shame.

FEMININE WISDOM AND RITES OF PASSAGE

In ancient times, sensuality was taught by the elders and wise Women of the tribe. The Higher Priestesses were chosen as girls coming into woman hood and guided how to carry this wisdom. They were the keepers of the feminine wisdom to prevent it from being manipulated and used as control and power. Girls entering their first blood phase of womanhood, were taught about sensuality, ways to honour their bodies, and how to teach a man the wise ways of sensuality and pleasure. The was a magical and very healing ritual where they were held in the highest honour, where touch was received by the other women, their own mother present for the ritual. During this ceremony, the girl entering womanhood her hymen was gently broken with a sapphire crystal and she would experience a whole-body orgasm of bliss. Sensuality was a magical celebration, and her blood flow was offered back to Mother Earth, as a gift of the feminine. This wisdom is being passed on and more men are becoming aware of it and its sacredness. May this feminine empowerment be a part of this collective shift. There is wise power within the menstrual flow of a woman, and a time when she reaches maturity and her menses cease to flow, her wisdom held within, as a wise woman at the prime of her sensual power. This woman was revered with the highest of honour.

The more we can each honour Mother Earth (Gaia), the more we are assisting in healing the collective of the feminine wound. With more becoming aware of the illusions and the deceit fed on a daily basis then the separation within this global collective is inevitable as timelines present. The cosmic intensity was felt in early 2019 and the transition from 2020-2021 saw a surge within humanity. This is not about making more noise; this is about exploring the transformational inner work.

It is time for each to rise up, be the change, and to empower the next generation with your fearless Feminine Rising.

THE LABELS/CAUSES

The only place for labels in on containers and bottles. This trilogy does not define me, nor does your story or journey define you. It refines you to honour and re-claim your inner truth! I keep morphing so I never play in a world of mediocrity, becoming adaptable and continuing to explore the unknown to evolve.

Some may have formed an opinion and label about me, from my story, life choices and the great part is, it's your opinion. An opinion is a great messenger to look deep inside to what you reject, fear and are learning to love. I have reached not caring, as to not live my path is suffocation itself.

I cannot deny that I used to feel hurt by what others thought of me, I wanted to be loved, liked and accepted by the tribe, to avoid feeling rejected; however, the training ground was perfect lessons to gain insight in how to live my truth. I am ready to take on the world stage. To be fully exposed, seen, up for public opinion as I know the power and the source wisdom that flows through me, is for the highest good. I know this to be The Feminine Source/God and I am loved no matter what. Nature will always bring inner peace as I live aligned with Natural, Universal and Spiritual Laws of the Universal Mother. I am loved and so are You.

We have found one another as Lighthouses for Humanity

We are walking one another home.

We are standing for the Children.

Freedom and Equality

I hear your truth

Really, I do,

Yet you forget

Like others do

That you chose this life

Before this time

That's right to experience

Variety over time,

What did you learn?

Are you staying stuck in your shit?

Are you willing to play the game?

Your Soul has a mission

To burry, wounds of hate,

Stand up for your rights

Before it's too late!

To let go of what was

To let go of your hate

To stop giving your power away

That seals your fate.

I'm not here to persuade you,

More inspire my truth

A lasting impression

To wake up our Youth

The children remember

Yet get entangled with drama

Your momma and Poppa

Both living their Dharma

You chose it

That's right

Your colour of your skin

Your religion too

An illusion of separation

hiding within!

It's falsely created

Not true you see.

Your flavour of sexuality

Tastes sweeter than thee,

Sensual pleasures

Sensuality is neutral

You know?

Fuck labels that stink

Of indifference and lack

Bullshit excuses keeping you stuck

Even entrapped, fancy that!

Let's make love over fighting

Have orgasms for humanity

and world peace too.

You can choose to resist it

Or join in with the fun?

Make mockery out of freedom

You each have a choice,

I shall state is fearlessly,

So, what's it to be?

Infinite love and Sovereignty?

A healthy expression.

No longer held bondage

In fear and repression!

When you're covered in crap it is hard to see,

The rough-cut diamond,

Staring back as me,

Transformed into the diamond,

Of limitless possibilities

All Shiny and glowing

No longer within an ocean of lack.

Willing to stand fierce in Your truth,

Within the crowd surrounding.

One drop of love enters their pond

A new time and reality

awakens above and beyond.

Still raw and authentic

And glowing with Love,

Fuck the labels of indifference

I see you staring back at me,

Your love rests within,

We are one harmony.

One step at a time,

No going back as we are here to shine

I walk here beside you

The place for labels is on bottle you see,

Fuck racism and hate,

And dissolve inequality.

Simply open your heart and

Feel into your soul.

A New Earth waits,

Freedom needs no approval

It is all from within

A revolution of Love.

Stop boxing yourself in,

Get up and love freely.

Stand up for Global Peace

Unified as ONE harmony

Freedom to express

Diverse sensuality, if you dare!

We are the truth

The leaders of change

Don't you see, you and I

A new Earth of equality,

So, put down the labels

And honour your Truth.

Swallow your pride and

Taste some humility

There is no separation,

That's fear you see

I love you my brother

I love you my sister

Across land and Sea

We are one and together

Till one day you will see

The only truth is equality

It is awakened within.

CHAPTER 2: SOUL JOURNEY

"I embrace the journey of opening my heart and the letting go of all that binds it" - Trudy Vesotsky

TRAPS & FREEDOM

Society will create rules and beliefs to keep others trapped, the veil of the illusion attempting to keep You in judgment. Sensuality has been dirtied up, feeding off animalistic repressed desires and feeding off a low toxic vibration. Your thoughts are like the sacred seeds of what you will create in your life, and must be protected from all negative influences, as any doubt will destroy their potency. Be courageous to follow the course, as you learn how to go with the flow and keep stepping up into who you came here to be. As mentioned in Breaking Free, society likes to control the masses. Here are the 3 main traps of repression that bind you in fear, anger and doubt.

- *Shame*
- *Blame*
- *Guilt*

This never-ending inward journey is a process of *'checking-in'* to witness where you fall back into shame, blame, guilt and fear of being seen. The traps are an illusion that keep you stuck in your rightness and wrongness of another. The media is filled with stories, public opinion thrives off them, and they exist within each and every soul lurking in the shadows. The judge hides behind and within the fear! It is with awareness that you unveil your unconsciousness and restore consciousness which is love. This does not happen overnight as we are creatures of habit and social conditioning.

Right thinking replaces wrong thinking with consistent awareness, until the upgraded thinking is re-wired. Feel into the heart and commit to rewiring the mind. Master Your inner world behind the veil to explore self-actualisation, self-realisation, the path of knowing thy self. Let's explore what assists shifting the blocks to access freedom.

DOUBT

Doubt is the greatest block of all, a lack of belief in Self and giving your power away to outside opinion. Don't be afraid to follow your heart and bliss as you fear others may judge you. Put that shit down as it plays on the strings of your unworthiness, helplessness and hopelessness. You didn't come here to shrink!

Know that there is an inner knowing that without a shadow of a doubt you will find your way as the path will reveal. There is always a way. No matter how long the path or inner struggle is, never giving up on you. Others may never believe in you, as they never have believed in themselves. Look doubt in the face and walk away from it. It has no place and will block your *Soul Codes* from being revealed. It is the jail cell that keeps you trapped. You have to shift belief into knowing and have faith in life improving. Doubt is no longer welcome!

Find a way, be hungry and go after it. It is your Souls destiny, and all doubt will block the view. Doubt is there to test your Faith in God.

FORGIVENESS

The inner critic is nosier than what others see, and it interchanges masks to hide as what is happening on the inside is a different story to what is shown to the world. If you are beating up on you, begin to see with fresh and rested eyes and be kind and loving to you. Begin to witness each perceived imperfection with love as forgiveness requires personal responsibility, a path to feel free. It is the inner thoughts and consequent behaviours that requites refining, not the person. This may be a massive hurdle, and personally it took me many years to shift beyond resentment. Emotional debris may be so deep that is has to be shifted by a professional who works with energy and the unseen in the auric field.

The one who is willing to go knee deep in thick mud and explore beyond what is comfortable. Ownership of self is empowering and the ability to ask for forgiveness builds trust, humility, love, compassion and Soul freedom.

If another is not ready to forgive you, then forgive self. Stop waiting as you may be waiting in vain. It was something in the past and it is time to put it down with love.

It is not your fault; it is okay to feel the pain and to know that you are loved. It is no longer relevant in the now, unless you keep entertaining it.

Allow your choices to be your own choices even when others may not approve remember it is none of anyone else's business. Make choices that bring no harm to the other with the knowledge you have at the time and chose what is aligned with your soul path. Own it and walk your most *aligned path.*

COMPASSION

As a child you had compassion for all living beings and nature. If you saw another upsetting another you would go to assist with no hesitation as naturally caring Souls. This is instinctual inner standing that overflows in compassion and love. Then, as the child develops a sense of identity and separateness, this is mine is learnt, and this is mine and the beginning of learning to establish boundaries. The transition to no longing wishing to share your toys and the identity of the entity as the individual. The challenge is when this is hardwired into adulthood and the fears unaddressed. Compassion is remembered when we soften outward judgement towards others and learn how to attend to the inner critic. Compassion walks alongside love. The more love for self, the greater your ability to be loving and compassionate towards others. To have compassion is to have deep understanding with gentleness, kindness, and forgiveness. It is the ability to see ourselves in others as we are all *perfectly divine reflections.*

To see the oneness in all Souls it begins with having courage to look within, to begin self-love, forgiveness, and experiencing the magic of aloneness.

HONESTY

When there is honesty and trust present within a relationship, love can flourish. This type of relationship is healthier than one with many rules. Too many rules lead to lies, shame, guilt, and an unwillingness to be honest. Honesty begins with being honest with self, your thoughts, feelings, emotions and choices. Honesty, requires vulnerability, and a willingness to be seen in your raw essence.

Your unique Soul path may not fit into what society conforms to and your path to learning to trust intuitive wisdom and stand proud in your own soul direction will reveal the more you evoke and listen to it.

The journey of honesty can easily shift into embarrassment which then becomes the liar. The aspect of self will hide behind a lie rather than be found out. The moment the Liar tells the lie, guilt stands at the door. Guilt begins to make the liar feel uncomfortable, until it becomes so unbearable, honesty can see the liar squirming. This happens in relationships; What's wrong? The response, 'Nothing!' Which is another lie where guilt becomes a heavier load. This will weigh the souls down leading to feeling depression and losing confidence, in Self.

Many of you have a fear of being rejected as when you shared your deepest fantasies in the past you were judged, told you were dirty, disgusting or called a slut. Your fantasies are your own deepest and darkest aspects of the pleasure mind, and I view them as sacred place. When another invites you into their deepest aspects of mind, you are a guest, so behave like one. It is not your business if you approve or not, or even to seek approval off your partner. It takes one of you to receive the other with unconditional love, no matter what is said and to remain present, open, and listen. With courage honesty will tell the truth. This will set the liar free.

Suppression of desires will create deviance, guilt and shame as this creates a toxic environment which is the perfect elixir for disease and illness. Be unapologetically you and be honest as it is a choice of the other how your truth is received. I have been told I can be cutting as in blunt, this may be true to the one receiving and yet, when instinct is clear then don't prolong the suffering by drawing something out. Life moves fast as you can stay bound in heaviness or meet the lessons like a badass warrior and restore gentleness.

HUMILITY

Be willing to own your emotions and reactions. To me humble means being able to be honest, admit your moments of unconsciousness and arrogance. To own your choices and desires as no one is perfect. Humility takes courage to see the other without biting or fighting back. The one who is humble has a great attitude, happy and full of laughter, never reacting to anything anyone says. When the ego kicks in, the rightness or wrongness of opinion, then humility has been left in the wake. The ego shifts very rapidly into arrogance when it is exposed. Arrogance will take everything personally, the ego becoming self-centered, entitled and unbearable to be around. Arrogance will butt in and will not allow the other the space to express.

Arrogance is the darkness of humility; it is angry at everything and has forgotten how to be humble. Gratitude is a way to be free. When arrogance kicks in, ask the ego to sit the f#ck down, be silent in your opinion and choose five-nice things to think about the person in front of you. The self-centered anger will begin to have less hold on you, and humility will return. Laughter will follow as you will see the ridiculousness of it all. Life is about stumbling and leaning into life.

When you mistake your judgement, you fall flat on our face and can get back up wiser and humbler. It is called being human and living the joy of life.

NATURE AND INTUITION

Nature holds the keys to connect with nature spirits and will accelerate the ability to allow intuition to come through. It is a place to remember the Spirit and soothe the Soul. There is stillness and the only noises are that of the natural elements, and many times children's laughter. There is also the nature within, a magical garden within each and every one of us, with a secret garden, we each hold the key to go there. The connection outdoors connects us to our inner world of Spirit and the garden of Eden. Book time each day to get out in nature, place your hands on the trees, your feet upon the Earths flesh and see what wisdom flows through and into you. Have gratitude and let in the love from the Earth's core and the higher dimensional beings within the crystal realms beneath your feet.

The more time you spend in nature, the greater your intuition comes through. It is challenging for intuition to be heard when there is much noise in the head and the external shit show of the media performance. Nature can yield to your command and holds the keys to your awakening and remembering.

The Angelic Realm

I am blessed to work with the Angelic energy. Some may get lost here and that is okay, as this may not be for everyone. Energy is energy and this is sensed and felt more than words. You get to choose what you invite in and what you chose to reject. The beautiful part is, once I invited the angelic in and was began using this with others, they never leave, and their presence grows stronger each time.

I have been granted permission from the Angelic Realm to pay this forward and to evoke this with those I work with. This was guided to be transcribed in teachings and writings so that it is available to those who feel a resonance to it. They entrusted me with how to evoke, scribe and to allow the words to use be intuitively guided.

I have been instructed to make clear, this is for personal use only. This is not an invocation to then use on others, the Angelic beings were very clear about this.

Having said that I deeply honour and respect all those that have been working with this angelic energy for many years. This is powerful and international clients have felt this transmission via facetime and zoom sessions.

This is one of the techniques that I bring into *The Sacred Womb and Yoni healing for Women around releasing sexual trauma.* This is also great for men that have experienced sexual trauma or being fed off by the unhealed feminine. To begin, find a quiet place where you can sit undisturbed and be still. Repeat the following, reading out aloud.

"I call in the Arch Angel Jophiel

To join in the presence of (Your name)

I call forth a golden beam of liquid of light

Glowing in radiance and beauty

To flow in through the crown

PAUSE

Trickling down, illuminating the crown

A warm glow of love and light

Suspended lightness within the body

Flowing freely, soothing the mind.

PAUSE

Dripping and flowing down

Bathing the throat in golden light

Allowing this golden nectar

To cleanse my voice of truth

PAUSE

Flowing smoothly deep into the chest

Bathing the heart in golden angelic light

Lightness, glowing and feeling nourished

The warmth spreading across the chest

Front, back, side and side, the whole chest

Bathed in golden sparkly light.

PAUSE

Feel the lightness and gentleness

Like a reflective shimmering from heart to crown

Feeling safe and feeling loved.

I am beautiful and abundant

Thank you, Jophiel

For this golden light

For reminding me,

I am loved."

This is available to you whenever you chose to access this. There is no force or searching as the angelic energy will find you. All you have to do is ask to receive. You are each remembering, layers of numbness dissolve, and you learn by free-falling into the unknown with trust and faith.

There are light beings surrounding you and all you have to do is ask to feel their presence and you will know as you will feel goosebumps or chills.

Chapter 3: Protective Armour

> *"You are the key to communicate with Source God and the angelic realm. All is seen, all is loved. God is Source, you are God. Nothingness & everything. And all in-between."* -Zoe Bell

The Armour of the Heart

Many of you do not fear failure, you fear success or being seen. Owning your voice and taking responsibility for your life is paramount. You fear greatness and what others may think of you as you rise. There is an untapped Source power within you, that many in power will not want you to access, as then they can longer control you. They may be afraid as you are leaping into a direction they don't yet understand, leap anyway. The fear of success means all the attention is upon you, the good, the bad, the ugly, and society is blood-thirsty for the later. As you learn to love yourself with healthy self-esteem and confidence in your abilities, your brave heart will radiate pure love and you will emerge fearless of being seen.

When connecting to your hobbies and passions your Spirit is free to express and your childlike heart is open. Follow your creative joy as this will be your Soul Calling. In this act of service, the heart opens with a feeling of limitless freedom and unconditional love (translating to no conditions).

Your heart is a lifeline to your Galactic teachers and where your Spirit dances free alongside other Spirits that are free. It is the heart that leads the eternal dance to celebrate your beauty, peace and harmony here in Earth, as above-so below to be conduit for light to shine through as you dance the *Middle Way* on this path of ascension.

Sometimes you don't realise how lost you are until the cracks of chaos appear and chinks in the armour release and this is where the pain starts to flow out. The armour is there to protect your most vulnerable aspects, the heart. To allow love in means a willingness to be courageous and explore and express your deepest fears whilst being present to feeling it all. When the emotion hits you like a freight train, follow it and go into it as it is a key to address your fears to reveal the true You. Souls may come in superfast and leave even faster, all is as is as each interaction is a gift in refining your hearts most sacred vocabulary. The infinite you on the path of the one.

SCARS HOLD STORIES OF PAIN

Receiving touch is a magical doorway to begin to melt the armour of the heart and to reconnect to tissue that is scarred and often holding trauma. This healing process of touch allows the layers to begin to melt. This came into my awareness during my soul journey of learning to receive sensual and sacred touch. I learnt about the correlation between the breast tissue and the labia and also the correlation between the clitoris and the nipples.

This was the healing of my scar tissue and learning to love my once flat boyish muscular chest.

Here is a brief background which relates to many women. At the age of 30 – years old I underwent a Bilateral Breast Augmentation. I hated the size of my breasts as I felt like a boy and was bodybuilding at the time. Many of the girls had fake boobs and I wanted to feel sexy and womanly. My self-esteem was in tatters and the self-loathing and shame was my inner world of daily poison. I had been breast obsessed since around the ages of 6 years old. The surgery left hardened scar tissue around my left breast which felt un-natural. While being massaged, it came up that there was stuck energy around my heart and so there began some self-touch exercises and the layers started to release. I started to sob and realised that my natural breasts I had had were beautiful. I apologised for hurting and not loving my body and began to tell myself I was enough. This was in 2016. That night, I did some more heart healing with loving touches of my breasts and yoni and more tears started to flow. My breasts were crying out to be loved.

I had allowed men to grab them roughly, pulling and squeezing my nipple so hard that I yelped. All the softness to lovemaking ignored and it was time to own the part I played in the scene. My heart was suffocating, and I was craving healing from the inside out. I had used my breasts to manipulate men into guiltless pleasures as a sexual object of desire and if I am honest, I loved the attention I got for my breasts for many years as I was trapped in sexual objectification.

Rose oil was used for the heart, and I bought six roses, three of which were red and three were pinks. The same day I saw the numbers thirty-three, seven times! According to angelic messages, the number 33 represents the

Ascended Masters. I was being held, protected as I went through this vital release of letting go and loving me some more. The angelic entourage that walks alongside. I scattered two of the rose petals over the bed, lay around and on top of them and massages my breasts and labia while listening to a Heart Chakra healing, from on YouTube channel, at a frequency 314 Hz.

The heart is a sacred place of love, compassion and joy. To let go of the resistance and trust in this process takes courage, inner strength and is the most protected organ of all. Your heart is the most challenging and yet, infinite realm to open and I now live from the sacred heart, July 2021.

The heart is protected by the casing of the ribs and chest bone and tissue takes time to soften with self-nourishment and with those I love dearly.

The breast massage is great to implement into your healing even when both breasts have been removed. Touch is vital for healing the individual using a figure-of-8 infinity pattern. The infinity sign is how the feminine Source energy flows in the body at each star portal. This is relevant for healing all scar tissue and a beautiful way to honour the beautiful Woman or Man that you are. This self-massage of the body continues to open up the vulnerable and courageous heart.

Life is about choices and free will and the consequences of the choice. This was my choice at the time, and I live with the consequences. I forgive myself for not honouring the magical beautiful petite breasts I was given. My heart is open to love and I embrace my breasts as they are, 20 years later. I have decided to explore 'Explant procedure' options, which is removal of bilateral breast implants. I feel a deep longing to return to my natural feminine state as my sensual essence is not based on the body. I feel healthy, lit up in my essence and asymptomatic. Recently, I have been healing the scar tissue with my quantum healing gifts and I feel more natural breast tissue emerging around the implants. Let's see what vibrational technology is being created across the globe by many brilliant Souls and see what doors opens as your universe always delivers the path.

VULNERABILITY

Your willingness to be seen in your rawest and deepest aspects of the soul, is an invitation to open your heart. The more you open the raw vulnerable aspects then the more you grow and evolve. Vulnerability cultivates presence which give other souls permission to open up. Now is a time of feminine manifestation and raw vulnerability which is a doorway to be walked through by both men and women. Believe it or not vulnerability is sexy and powerful when you shift beyond the story. This is not about crying all the time either, this is the willingness to be courageous and honest and express from your brave heart. As a woman it is vital to allow your man to be a man in his true essence, so male bonding with other males is important and not speaking over his voice or shaming his emotions.

Here is an example of the power-play of these energies between couples, and the way that nature will re-polarise.

This is was aspect of two on-line programs that I created and ran for 3-years: The Divine Masculine and The Divine Feminine Blueprint. I still guide souls through one to one or within a retreat setting.

A woman may push and push her partner until he snaps at her, raising his voice, it is as if unconsciously she desires to feel his raw masculine energy. Hearing him raising his voice is the fire. Now, she feels his raw masculine energy of passion coming through, she crumbles and yet on a deep level is turned on. For many, this may be hard to comprehend. He may respond after she breaks down in tears as there is a window of opportunity for healing. The recovery that can follow, may include him expressing his emotions, of how much he loves and cares for her. They both have one another's unwavering presence. Their collective energies are magnetically charged, and a re-polarisation has occurred, as she has dropped back into the feminine of receiving. Primally drawn to one another, what concludes is a very passionate embrace of make-up sex and deeply connected lovemaking.

With the balance restored everything runs smoothy until the next rules are placed upon the relationship. A power-struggle between the sexes is an unhealthy way to control and manipulate the other, and all rooted in insecurity and fear. This is for both the man and the woman. This is a reason behind many relationships going pear-shaped, full of rules or the childish threats of the ultimatums. Like, seriously.

Vulnerability requires looking into the shadows of your fears and to explore the inner journey to the I am Soul. All fears stem from insecurity. The three things that will shift these a full 180 degrees in consciousness are daily rituals to nourish You.

- *Self-love, self-worth and letting go of the need to control.*

It is not your inability to trust others, it is the fact you are unable to trust yourself. Deep within there is something you have been unwilling or afraid to love, accept and forgive within. You will do anything so that your fears or secrets are not found out and this is the basis of why many tell lies.

- *In each relationship You are each the perfect reflection of one another*

Having too many rules will lead to disappointment and one party either bending to meet all needs or rebelling against the rules. It is really vital to have open communication at the beginning of any relationship, so that you both know what you will and will not accept. There is never any need to control another, the only things you can ever learn how to control are your own thoughts, your breath and your reaction to the external world around you. The rest is none of your business.

- *Love is unconditional and free to express in divinity.*

COURAGE AND TRUST

The ability to wake- up and evolve is determined by the extent of your awareness and the willingness to let go of the old of what you think you know or are holding onto. This creates an expanded way of being, seeing and living with one another.

This pathway takes courage, trust, compassion and loving kindness. There are no mistakes in life and many pathways to explore off track to learning as we each grow into the *'middle way'.*

It is the rightness and wrongness of the other that will keep you trapped in the old matriarchal and patriarchal way of being that has been imprinted in your psyche. I am still learning and growing and that is the magical beauty and offering of life and not knowing what is coming, is exciting! I know it is big and I am ready to absorb it all, now that the foundational tools are fully integrated into my being, no matter what happens, I will always allow my creative expression to run-free and come back to Self as a lone wolf and still scream into a pillow or out in the wild.

That is your true power, Source and God Self.

FAITH

Faith is trusting in a force greater than you can currently see. Faith never leaves you as it is forever waiting within. Faith is your ability to follow the signs upon your path, and to know that the Universe has your back. Each twist, turn and pause present as an access point to reach the highest version of you. At the time you may not understand why something is happening as there is a bigger picture at hand. Faith requires trusting in a higher power within and without you. God, Source, Consciousness and what other names you wish to give it.

This requires trusting and having faith in the unknown.

HONOURING THE DIVINE FEMININE

This is a powerful process to dissolve the protective shell and a pathway to nourish the feminine insides and be held with unconditional love by the divine masculine. The feminine is your creative, playful, imagination and free in all aspects of the soul and she is within each of our great men.

The Shamanic ceremony was held in a swimming pool, where I was guided, held and supported by a fellow Shaman, a beautiful dear friend of mine. I was given medicinal mushrooms to assist in creating a fresh loop to weave into my upgraded reality. A low dose was used thus creating an inner environment of being more connected with nature within and without. The focus was not on creating a hallucinogenic tripping your ass off response.

This has to be experienced to fully reap the rewards and was a key to dropping into the feminine and allowing layers of unconscious tension of the wounded masculine to dissolve. The water, feminine in nature with a magical sensual feel against the skin. I was held floating, lovingly guided by the divine masculine.

This is led by a Shaman or Soul that has the capacity to hold sacred space and a grounded container that supports the healing, meaning divine presence during the entire ceremony. During these ceremonies, the shaman will be using the same plant medicine as to open up into higher dimensions and to assist in weaving the dreaming.

The pain and trauma are like hidden blocks of armour held under the skin, and deep in the tissues. The release happens as the environment creates trust, faith and leaning into unconditional love. By giving the body time to relax with no force these aspects are given the honour they deserve bringing each individual into a state of healing.

This takes the individual into a deeper connection with the sensual and feeling body and immersed in the water adds a potency. The sensual feminine caress of water, a holy ceremony and a re-birth into your freer skin. Sensuality of waters fluidity is lifegiving and water has a powerful healing tonic on the body, mind and Soul. The water has to be contained as in a shallow pool or spa for safety reasons and to keep the space contained, sacred and supported in all ways.

I have been guided that it is where I am assisted by the spirit realm. The water is magical for healing work of the womb space and divine feminine. This is relevant for both the biological woman and the biological man. This may open the blocks around the relationship with mother and father and providing an opportunity to melt the blocks of protection around the heart.

When a divine woman is held and rocked by the sacred masculine with words expressed with loving kindness deep heart healing takes place. The words expressed were, 'everything is okay'. In this simple expression, layers of protection of the wounded inner masculine begin to drop away. The resistance came up, another layer ready to dissolve, the tears bubbled up and deep emotions released. Silence and the orchestration by nature, pure presence with the eyes and a deep and very safe connection. A feeling of being held by the protector, the sacred masculine. This is where emotions and memories of my dad came up, and lifetimes healed.

Following the process in the water, I was guided to a room, lay onto the bed, naked, and began to anoint my own body with oils. A mix of macadamia, ylang -ylang and rose oil. The scent and oils of the Goddess Isis and Queens. I was given space to drop deeper within, and following some deep relaxation was joined by my beautiful friend. I received healing touch and inner healing of deep surrender as I was honoured as the divine feminine by the guidance of the sacred masculine. Words cannot describe what transpired and a memory of love forever etched upon my heart and soul.

The next day, my skin smoother and softer and different. My entire bodysuit upgraded and restored to lightness and pure innocence. I looked softer and more relaxed in the face. The joy of life oozed from my being. I felt free and reborn.

I have since guided couples through this in 1:1 setting and forecast this in up-coming retreats.

Here is a way to 'do it yourself', a process to explore honouring the divine inner masculine. These are the aspects once hidden, shammed and dishonoured. This is also the protector that did not have its voice of NO honoured or heard as a child. This can be something so simple as the defiant 3-year-old that knows exactly what he or she wants, not feeling heard. It is a vital aspect in the development of the child and can lead to the programs of the damsel in distress and in men the knight in shining armour.

This is an aspect of the woman that holds up her sword up in protection and is pushing many great men away. It is time for the inner masculine to heal and rest its sword down for the divine connection with the masculine. Ladies, never stop expressing your truth and if you are cut down mid speech then bring your divine masculine out and express your fearless truth. As when you express it is like an atomic bomb of raw sensual passion and sage wisdom.

- *This is a step- in healing humanity.*

It is now time for you to heal. Following this healing we shift into honouring the inner child, once lost, silenced and for many forgotten.

HONOURING THE DIVINE MASCULINE

- Stand up and read out loud, own it, and keep repeating.

"I honour the inner masculine as much as my inner feminine, an aspect I shamed and ignored, kept away in the dark. I release all blame, and guilt. I will listen to you and honour your voice to be heard. I will be honest with all sensual and sexual desires. I shall see no wrongness of your deepest thoughts and fantasies.

If you fuck up, I will forgive you right away, as you made a choice, and there will be no more punishment. No matter what, I am always here for you. I will endeavour to be always open, and I release all non-logical emotions. I love you and thank you for being my protector as it is time to rest your sword down"

HONOURING THE INNER CHILD

Your inner child holds the key to the inner sparkle and passion that ignites your Soul path- This is within my third book *'Completeness- a doorway to love.'*

I invite you to spend some quiet time alone exploring these next few questions of self-enquiry. The intention is to shine the light of truth to gain clarity into what you are being or wanting to be.

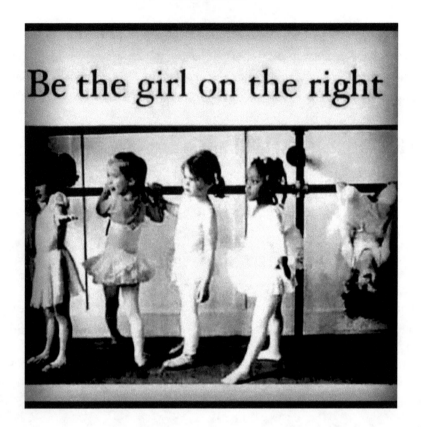

Think back to when you were five or six, even 3 years old.

- What did you love to play with?
- What are the things you did?
- What was your natural state of being?

Now ask yourself.

- Does that sound like the things I am passionate about?
- What makes me happy?
- What do I love to read? – Are they all related?

If that is really challenging.

- What would it feel like to be five or six again?
- What does it look like?
- What did you dream of doing and being?
- Did you dress up, and as what?
- And whom did you aspire to be like?
- Who inspires you today and why?

This is a fun and powerful exercise as it holds many keys to what you came here to do as Soul. Never forget, the only person holding the key, is you!

No Excuses

If money was unlimited

What would you be?

Your scars dissolved

Infused, a fresh possibility.

What would you be?

Imagine a state

Free from the judgment

And free from hate

A self-created insanity

A distorted reality

A bullshit excuses

Now, who is the Muse?

Imagine being five or six

Unlimited imagination

Not giving a shit

No longer a hostage of

Your mind of bullshits

PROTECTIVE ARMOUR

A victim of your circumstances

Who cares?

Stop blaming

Cursing and pointing

Fuck that negative shaming!

Start to dream a bit

And keep building your vision

Everyday commit to grow

Come apart in tears

Make getting up your mission,

Repeat and never give up!

Be inspired

To follow your bliss

Ducking and weaving

Others fucked up bullshit.

Your choices and dreams

You're newfound reality

Be the change, it's all awaiting

No more excuses

You are lovelight and light love

As the only real fight is within

Work on your vibe

Call out to your tribe

People that inspire you

To love you

And guide you.

Never to catch doo-doo again

To hold you accountable

As you grow and explore

To reveal your divinity

Raw authenticity

Rare beauty blossoming

And never ever be

Hidden within, again.

Z

CHAPTER 4: UNIVERSAL MAGNETISM

"I don't care that they stole my idea...I care that they don't have any of their own." – Nikola Tesla

A MAGNETIC FORCE

Your spine is the antenna to the outside world, as is every hair on your body. When your spine is out of alignment, your health, vitality and energy are impacted. This will affect outcomes in life, be it success or failures. Life is a series of lessons of contrast and consequences of your choices, frequency and the polarity of the invisible substance within and around you.

The body is one huge magnet as everything in the Universe has poles. Everything has a pair of opposites. Opposites are identical, but different in degree. All paradoxes are explained by an understanding of this Principle. Polar opposites are half-truths of the whole truth.

Have you noticed how you feel some mornings when you get out of bed, you feel like you've had a workout and your body feels scrunched up and tight? It feels like it's been hit by a truck and if your neck is affected then your energy feels drained. Perhaps your emotions (the 7- dwarfs) are grumpy and tired. You feel like you have been plugged into the dream matrix, where you spend your dreamtime doing mission work like Neo and Trinity? This is exactly what happens, like getting plugged into your subconscious to clear up and do the Cosmic work in your dreamtime state. I am planting a seed of curiosity, and before I take you down a rabbit hole let's get back to the topic of magnetic force.

By moving, stretching and shaking your body, you will start to wake-up the Prana (ether), which fills all space, solids and gases as it is static in nature. You start an inner activation and excitability within every cell of your body. Diving deeper in your spinal cord there is a canal running either side of the spine and within the substance of cerebral-spinal fluid there is a negative and positive current of human electricity running through your body.

This has an impact on your health, prosperity, longevity and magnetism to the outside world. It is this fluid that contains the electrical current which is fluid and kinetic. The body is magnetic so will have both a positive and negative pole. The positive pole on the right-hand side of the body is called Pingala and the left side of the body Ida and they start at the right and left nostrils.

The air passes into the nostrils, through the interior canal of the nose, passed the pharynx, the larynx, the windpipe, the bronchial tubes and enters the lungs. The oxygen passes across the cellular membrane mixing with the blood and it is from here that combustion takes place. As the blood takes up the oxygen, it exchanges carbonic gases to be expired into the outside world.

It is when the natural magnetic properties within the vessel cease to absorb or radiate energy, from and to the surrounding space, its magnetic properties cease.

This is called being dead.

Humans can go months without food, weeks without water, minutes without oxygen and yet, not even a nano-second without this vital life force energy. These negative and positively charged poles cross through each of the energy wheels known as the Chakras/Energy wheels/Star Portals. The energy absorbed and radiated will differ depending on if it from the positive or negative poles. These energy junctions /wheels are impacted by the thoughts that you are having as each emotion creates a specific charge and magnetic vibratory charge. Now add that into the equation that each pole will radiate a different charge and you are looking at some serious alchemy and at times chaos!

Have you ever had that feeling when someone has walked into the room, they are magnetic, and you feel drawn to them? You have to moved towards them and you feel this deep resonance with them, even a strong attraction. It may not be the physical that you are attracted to it may be their sexual magnetic field and radiance of their nervous system.

'I am part of a light, and it is the music. The Light fills my six senses: I see it, hear, feel, smell, touch and think. Thinking of it means my sixth sense. Particles of Light are written note. O bolt of lightning can be an entire sonata. A thousand balls of lightning is a concert. For this concert- For this concert I have created a Ball Lightning, which can be heard on the icy peaks of the Himalayas' - Nikola Tesla

Let's explore the different characteristics of these energies which acts as the 3- channels within the body-mind energy light-field.

THE CHANNELS OF THREE RIVERS

- Ida is the Yin- Feminine energy channel
- Pingala is the Yang - masculine energy channel
- Sushumna – The central channel.

Beyond biology you each have masculine and feminine energy channels.

Learning to work with the polarities are key.

Here are the different characteristics between them.

IDA

- Yin- Feminine- The left nostril- Moon- Creativity- Imagination
- Truthfulness- Kindness- Reverence- Spirituality- Fear- Timidity
- Parasympathetic Nervous system- Sleepy- Mental energy.

PINGALA

- Yang- Masculine- Right nostril- Sun- Determination- Drive

- Martial *"fighting spirit"*- Unusual aggressiveness- Strength
- Sympathetic nervous system- Energising- Physical energy.

The canal within your spinal cord is called Sushumna and this is the space where there is Unification of the physical (masculine) and mental (Feminine) energies. This Pranic energy is Omnipresent vital energy of the Cosmos, within Man and the entire material Universe. This life-force energy is said to be of two forms, physical and mental energy.

Feminine Rising in Consciousness means working with the Magnetic forces of the Sacred waters and inner Fire.

The upward awakening of allowing the Kundalini to rise is through practices of breath work, movement, bodywork, meditation, spine alignment and the foods you eat. These assist to attain higher states of Consciousness of the Christ Consciousness.

This polarity of forces can also lead to a downward spiral of the Kundalini energy of unrestrained lust and death

The Kundalini energy lays dormant sleeping at the base of the spine, known as Mooladhara. This is the Sanskrit term of the 1st chakra, energy wheel also called a Star portal, which connects us all to Mother Gaia, upon the redness of the Earth and to remember your Mission to Serve and honour the Earth beneath you.

The Root that keeps You and I plugged into the Earth Star, to be a conduit between the Earth and Cosmos.

The Kundalini is called the "Tree of Knowledge"

This is a path to the Garden of Eden, the Tree of Life and Samadhi 'Bliss consciousness' and the Awakened Earth where Heaven is a place within upon Earth.

It is the path to eternity and by accessing these portals replenishes as the *Fountain of Life.* The Kundalini is Two Serpents coiled sleeping until the conditions present to arise naturally with the birthing of the Golden Child (Innocence).

Let us celebrate the magnetic Mother forces of the feminine as we continue to explore the light and dark edges of inner healing to rise in grace and glory. The rising is the mother, also known as IDA, the feminine moon and the allowing this remembrance of wisdom and to trust in the process is to trust that GOD/Source exists. Give it all over to God and the truth of God, which is consciousness in divine expression.

The One creator and You are a divine reflection manifest. Remember what the HU-man is as the manifestation of man as the light of God.

The journey and adventure of life is to come into balance and harmony and learn how to work with the polar opposites within you and without you and come into Unification. The Divine Union is where the thoughts and emotions align and the manifestation with intentional action as the Golden Child. To know they Self is to know the Universe. The golden child is the returning of innocence as the curious explorer of the unknown.

The Divine union is not about seeking it within another, this is why there is a society of codependent humans bound in their excuses and fear of being alone and thinking they are only half complete when alone. True inner power comes when each individual has come into union with all aspects of self, the divine feminine and divine masculine as the golden child.

In the beingness of your radiance you will have brought to you by magnetic attraction who and what is next within your field of Spiritual growth. True human evolution is by relating to one another. The bond is through the heart and love. Consciousness is love and this is where you and I are here to evolve beyond the fear and be the embodiment of light, a cup overflowing in infinite love.

It is why women and men were created the way they were, there is a divine plan why we fit the way we do and sexual union of man and woman within a love frequency in full transparency. This trust of self is a key for human kin to survive.

Your body is a gift of raw sensuality, and you are the Holy Temple for the Holy Spirit to express as a Divine creative expression of harmony.

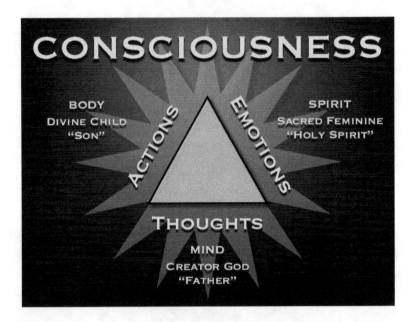

Mind- Body & Spirit

This diagram will become more relevant as a reference point as you go through the book and to integrate into your moment-to-moment choices in life. This is taken from *The Natural Law* presentation by Mark Passio.

Natural Law and Spiritual Laws of the Universal Mother I was intuitively guided along my path. The Knowledge presented after the direct experiences of learning through my journey called life to reinforce the path least travelled, and to know I was on track. There are no coincidences only consequences, synchronicities and truth.

A SUPERPOWER WITHIN

As soon as you hear the word Superpower, what do you think of?

Wonder Woman, Superman, and even Superhuman? There are many superpowers that you have, and you have simply forgotten how to access them. Life lessons and pathways are bringing opportunities to accelerate your growth, consciously and unconsciously and some areas of the brain are not being accessed. Some are chasing the golden egg, and forget their own eggs that need daily love, protection and attention until they are hatched. The golden egg is within You as the golden child. This is like your gifts, it is not something you get as each is revealed when you are ready to address your fears and move deeper into the shadows, pain body and emotional body.

It is time reveal what is keeping you stuck. Perhaps you are feeling in a rut of worn-out excuses and apathy. Is now a good time to release the blocks that sound like, *I don't want this, and why is life so unfair?*

I was blind, and now I see.

I was scared, and now I am brave.

I was numb, and now I feel.

I was courageous to explore, beyond the Veil.

I became lost, so I ventured beyond.

Trust and Faith developed as wings.

I know as you are reading this you will be upgrading in your vibratory field, as each word is coded with light to activate and inspire you to take action on the opportunities presenting in your life. Perhaps you are done with the manilla vanilla life, and as when you see others living in a world of abundance, opportunity and expansion, your cells in your body get excited. I am not talking about material stuff, I am referring to being internally rich and oozing with life force that life becomes lighter and simplified, and abundant with love. It is then that your greatest life flows to you.

Let's see what a cause is and why it attracts the unwanted.

YOUR INNER NAVIGATION SYSTEM

There is a tiny piece of brain matter that houses a bundle of nerves at your brainstem that filters out all the unnecessary information, so the real important stuff gets through. This is known as The *Reticular Activating System*. When you set a focus on (Goal – action of intention) what you want, then the RAS creates a filter for it, sorting and sifting through data, so only the relevant pieces that are important are brought to your attention and awareness. This all happens without your conscious awareness of it. It is the reason for getting what you don't want as that is your focus, oops!

It is your beliefs that will shapes your perception of reality as the RAS seeks information to validate your beliefs. It is the reason you learn about something and then you see it everywhere as it is in your conscious awareness. It was there all the time; you simply had no active awareness of it.

Take an example of experiencing jealousy or being suspicious of your partner. The RAS will begin to show you situations that are aligned with your thoughts to reinforce the belief, which is a lie you tell yourself. It will give you what you believe to be true. Even complaining about being late for work, you will create more things to be late for, as this is your focus. This is how the magnetic field of thought plays out and why rewiring the mind begins to address the cause.

You get what you focus and think about all the time

- Change happens at a subconscious level, by focusing upon a goal.
- Think of the situation/goal, you wish to influence & impact now.
- Think about and feel into the situation and goal and feel it deep within your entire body and the emotions you feel.
- See yourself in the picture, the movie as if it is playing out in the future, all happening in this now.
- Take note of the sounds, conversations and your visual surroundings.

See yourself in it as if it is already happening as everything is in the now.

- Book time in everyday, to daydream and visualise your movie. That way the conscious mind gets to play, and the realm of the subconscious mind 'imagination' gets to play together.

- Your imagination is powerful as the Creator God "Father"
- The RAS will be the power of influence of the world around you.
- It will bring the best solutions aligned with your goal and intention and this may be in experiences to learn from to refine you as the co-creator or destroyer of your life.

Welcome to a superpower that has your back and your best interest at heart. You get to change and create your future. Your past does not define you it was there to shape and refine your choices upon the path of self-mastery.

Distinguish between relevant and irrelevant information, the role in motivation and goal setting. Once this fires up with a right way of thinking about the wanted, the unwanted will begin to drop away.

It is like a 'bouncer' of information. It will let information through, so you recognise and respond to your name, and anything that threatened the safety of those you love and care for.

Each a lesson to learn more about who you are as Soul.

You cannot perceive what you are not in a vibration of
– Bashar-Darryl-Anka

The reticular activation system is similar to a GPS device and once you have planted a destination its job is to take you from where you are at A, to B. Once you become crystal clear on what you desire and set an intention, to achieve the goal, the RAS then it will activate and heighten your awareness. The idea is to let go of the vision as what you have as the vision may not be the greatest alignment that is coming to you, it may be playing a role to take you on the path as life has a rascally way of shifting the posts and presenting magical experiences along the way. See the world through the eyes of your curious and playful heart.

Be diligent to block out all things that are a distraction and nourish your powerful imagination.

Daily connection to your physical body, practices of the mind and connecting with passion that ignite your Spirit are key to your magnetic free-Queen-see. Shift your vibratory state to begin living in a state of flowing experiences. Follow your hearts greatest excitement until you can seek no further and drop in exhaustion and keep reaching for what brings the greatest excitement to your heart.

If you have never set an intention, the begin today, even if you are unclear on what you want, then chose to feel better than you do. For many, their minds are over-loaded with business, and the left-brain dominance. The practice of imagining, daydreaming, and having creative pursuits will stimulate the right-side of the brain.

As awareness increases and heightens the relevant information will be brought to you. Your own inner Genie!

THE POWER OF INTENTION

Without intention, there is no direction in life. You will have all experienced this, going along in life unconscious of your consistent thoughts and attracting more of the *'unwanted'*, The Law of Attraction. Intention is also the awareness of your direction and will align that which is tuned into the vibration of the intention. There are many in life who blame their current circumstance on life challenges and conditions, that are outside of themselves. The fact that they are single, and that all the great men and great women are taken, or that all the good ideas have been done and there is nothing left for them. This is a mindset of scarcity and will bring even more scarcity, so it is even more in their face. The more people complain about their life and the *'what's wrong with it'*, then guess what? The more they will receive exactly what they are complaining about! Be in a state of gratitude and observe what unfolds for you.

ABUNDANCE

The power of the RAS, intention and the breath impact your ability to attract success, wealth, health and abundance. It is a direct connection with consciousness. Like everything, discernment is required and to respect the right application of knowledge to support the individual with uploading higher levels of energy into the body vessel or meat body suit. Otherwise, it is like placing software into a computer that computer does not have the capacity or app to translate the signal and will blow the system out and this is why psychosis can kick in, as a safety *'deactivation'* switch until the Laya (veils of the mind) nervous system and body suit are ready to receive the higher frequency. It is why there are symptoms with the ascension, waking-up and upgrading process. If a body was to receive higher levels of love and peace that light beings emanated without a gradual process, then the human would combust and burst into flames. This is something I saw in my dreams and something I am guided to say, is a prescience.

Your greatest wealth is your health, as without your health how can you enjoy the fruits of the riches? Without adequate riches, then how can you access the availability to health? Both are inter-related.

- Are you beginning to see how you each have equal ability to create what you desire?
- You can attract the abundance of the wanted or unwanted. Abundance is abundance. So be mindful what you focus upon.
- Get rid of Tinder and dating apps once you tap into this. Indeed, it can be raining men, and raining women. You get to choose, and Universe will align what is best to assist you in your growth and that may be to have a dry spell to learn how to turn your Free Spirit on!

Your sensuality is part of this life-force, as by stirring the sensual awakening and during orgasmic states of pleasure are your most abundant states for creating in this heightened state of arousal just before you orgasm. Remember, you attract more of what you are consistently thinking about.

As you gain greater awareness of this energy you can learn how to move it around the body and direct it with the mind. This is to be used wisely and not to manipulate others as this is a sexual distortion seeking power and control. Learn how to explore the sensual energies in your body and how to replenish your energy levels naturally and in Self-governance as a sovereign being.

The Universal Law of Free Will symbol on the book cover will assist in lessons upon the Great Karmic Board of life. All to assist returning to unity, love and peace through a path of transcendence within a realm of transitions.

Chapter 5: The Body Principles

"Immobility is daily suicide" - Scott Sonnon

Movement

As mentioned prior your meat body suit requires flushing, moving, touching, massaging, stretching and marinating. Areas become blocked, emotions stuck, and old trauma lays stagnated for years. This stuck toxic energy gets deposited in the tissues of the body and this restricts you stepping into your full potentiality of fluidity and adaptability. The physical edges need to be free, flexible and malleable to change. To feel good on the inside you must radically shift your physiology and start working with the physical body. Let's look at this more tangibly so you can feel and ease into *The Art of Applied Action*.

- Sit slumped, hunched over and feel into your energetic state.
- Stay here for a while and see what emotions and sensations emerge.
- Now, sit upright, roll your shoulders and relax into your skin as if you are gently landing into your bodysuit for the first time.

- Shoulders are relaxed, belly relaxed, jaw relaxed and even the pelvic floor and anus relaxed.
- Notice your breathing and energy state in these two different positions.

- What did you notice and feel?
- If nothing, then explore it again and exaggerate it, work it to feel the differences in the energy states of your sensing experience.

You are a multilayered Spiritual being, and no matter who you are, the key is to start at the outer layer. Yes, the bits you can see, touch and feel. From the outside you move inwards much like pealing back the layers of an onion. There are tears that may release during these releases of stuck stagnant energy. The moments of being un-comfortable in a yoga posture that feels challenging and the discipline to be perfectly still and meet the resistance of the holding pattern. The key is to breathe into all places of resistance and avoid the temptation to move away from the posture too soon. This takes courage and you won't want to do it, initially. Once you get into it, you will begin to love it by the way you start feeling way more relaxed and even states of orgasmic bliss. When the body is ready to let go it will naturally make room for space and over time the tissues will become easier to work with.

'Change your physiology and you start to change the way you feel, change the way you feel inside, and you will give a different message to the world' – Zoe Bell

Mobility is great for taking all the joints through their full range of movement, in order to stay juiced, healthy and lubed. As lubrication is squeezed out by sitting and immobility- the joint loses its shock absorption ability, and this is why many get pain. Without that fluid you lose your ability to sense the world around you. The fluid holds the nutrition for the joint!! There is a surplus of infinite energy always within, a bright inner light that never fades, the energy is waiting to be un-leashed and expressed. As mentioned previously, your spine is an antenna connecting you to the outside world and impacts the frequency you emanate.

'That which is Above is like that which is Below. That which is Below is like to that which is Above. The Macrocosm (the very large: the totality) and the Microcosm (the very small: the individual units which comprise of the whole) are Reflections of each other. The Universe is Holographic: it is self-similar across all scales. This is *The Principle of Correspondence,* one of the General Principles of Natural Law.'

You are connected to the Cosmos and the Earth, a conduit for the Torus field of energy to flow through. You have to shake up the Cerebrospinal fluid that runs down the spine to bathes each of the energy wheels and vital glands with this high vibrational substance. This magnetic ocean of substance is designed to flow into the stagnation in the tissues and joints to retore fluidity beyond a suicide mission of immobility. This substance impacts vitality, health, magnetism and wellbeing.

By sitting at a desk all day, you have a time bomb of sickness. Writing a trilogy has weathered a storm or twelve in my body and I am now attending to my flexibility as my hips are screaming out. The Cosmic energy upgrades are felt firstly in the physical body of density with tightening of the joints and pain being the messenger to move, pay attention and learn to adapt. Stand more, begin daily mobility and hold yoga postures using gravity to

SOUL CODES

assist and explore the sensations within each movement.

Stretching, movement and balance are vital for evolution and functional longevity. Yes, the body speaks, and you are being eased into expansion and many teenagers have the most restricted and tight bodysuits of all due to the harmful environments of gaming, heavy school bags and postures that are screaming out to be stretched.

Here's why I say this with such conviction. When a joint lacks mobility that area loses the ability to move. Basically, you lube it, stretch it, or lose it. Pain is not the enemy it is the Spirit saying… *Hey (name), move me.... It's time to play!*

As lubrication squeezes out of the joints, the joints loose shock absorption ability. Not only do restrict your ability of fast response as a Warrior, but you also lose your primal ability to sense the environment (movement, position and force), all vital for the primal intuitive survival response for human evolution as the Superhuman. Worst of all, that fluid in the capsule between your joints holds nutrition and if you cannot move then you become the easy target or prey! Perhaps, now you will move and stop mutating into the walk dead of Zombies.

When you don't mobilise each joint daily, no matter how good your nutrition and water intake is, your connective tissue is literally starving because the nutrition you ingest is not being passed out to the areas that desperately need it. Your spine is vital to your energy levels, manifestation ability, magnetism and state of wellbeing. Yes, I am repeating myself as I is a vital key, take note and action.

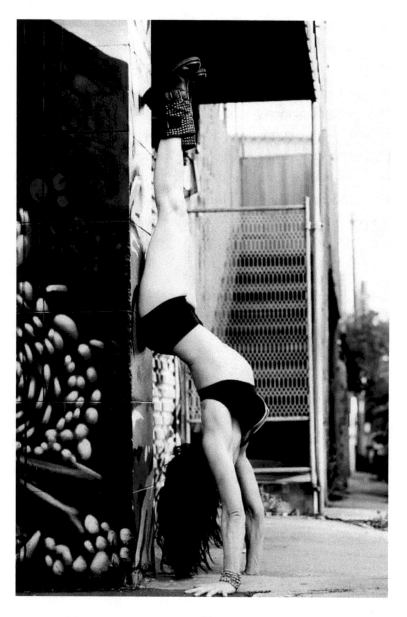

Play meets Yoga & Graffiti to weave and create

It is the law of the Universe that aliveness is defined as movement and death as stillness. From an emotional standpoint and a physical reality; mobility equals freedom, and immobility equal slavery. Humanity has been rapidly de-evolving rather than evolving. To become vibrant and evolve to a higher vibration of consciousness you have to adapt as the advanced species. You must move your body from simplicity to complexity every day. To play with balancing postures assists the evolving human to move with ease. This is not about pushing until you drop, that is the art of stupidity and a massive ego! Set a goal and aim a little below and continue to progress and build upon your achievements which gains momentum.

Restore and move your body to super charge with *Chugging or* dance

Chugging:

- Stand with your feet hip width apart
- Arms hanging loose- shoulders relaxed
- Keep toes on the earth and start bouncing up and down
- Only heals lift, arms floppy
- Bouncing up and down
- Body loose and free
- Exhale through a relaxed open mouth

Chug for 2-5 minutes

- Stand still- close the eyes and feel into the life force pulsating through the cells. This is what is it feel like to 'Be Lit & Alive'

THE BENEFITS OF MOVEMENT

- Wakes up all cells within the body.
- Removes toxins and waste from the body faster.
- Wakes up the energy in the sacral area, the energy centre related to sexuality and creativity.
- Healthier cells vibrating at a higher frequency- *'good vibes'*
- Wakes you up like a cup of coffee!
- Ability to maintain youthfulness and vitality and reverse the stiffening ageing process
- Tap into the Fountain of Youth- the *elixir of life.*
- Flush the joints with nutritious synovial fluid and bathe them with mobility to reduces joint pain.
- Increases flexibility and speeds recovery.
- No more pain in sexual positions if living with arthritis
- Calms the nervous system
- You will feel *sexier*
- Better *sex and orgasms* due to *increased flow to* the hips and pelvis.
- Confidently move from a powerless to a powerful state
- From **Fear to Flow** – the nervous system adapts – *to release fear* in the body with movement and the breath.
- *Prolonged sitting-* contributes to infertility, impotency, painful periods, low energy, sickness and difficulty orgasming.
- All blocks in the pelvis will restrict vital lifeforce flow of the sensual and healing forces of nature.

POSTURE OF CONFIDENCE

Your posture gives a strong statement to the world. How you carry and hold yourself will change the way you feel inside. Walking with effortless poise and the hips moving freely side to side is *sexy and healthy*, and a butt that has power in it. Learn how to move your hips with your heart lifted, and your head held high is a key to attraction as a badass that is not easy prey. Walking with your head hung low, shoulders slumped and a butt that is tucked under looks like a dog that is in shame. You become a target for sexual predators as you are giving of the vibration of shame and a victim. Get really clear on your thoughts, let go of what no longer aligns and be the one to align your frequency. Your posture and the way you choose to *move* will affect your energy within and thus, impacting life experiences and the opportunities that present.

Standing up tall is key as a human here to be a guiding lighthouse for others to find You. How will you radiate and reflect light of the 144,000 starlight portals within from a vessel that is unmalleable, stiff, slumped and unable to house the increase in the light energy?

The vessel is vital to strengthen, keep mobile and the ability to balance as this is also connected to the inner-ear and proprioceptive awareness to where the body is in space. Much is being lost within modern day living with feet encased in shoes adding to the disconnected in-authentic human, yes chakras/star portals of light within the feet, hands, fingers and through the whole body.

WATER & SALT

Your bodies are meant to be 70-80% water, and for some this is way lower. Alarm bells are ringing in the cells as this is a way to age faster like a shriveled-up prune. Water moves in a cyclical pattern, so mobility drills, Martial Arts and Tai Chi type movements take each joint through full ranges of movement. Many bodies are dehydrated, and many are drinking poor quality water laced with *fluoride* that their body % maybe closer to 60-65%. That is scary and also related to *women not getting naturally aroused sexually and may impact erections and sperm mobility in men.*

Water conducts energy within the sea of substance of both a negative and positive charge. Your emotions act as waves of sound and your thoughts act as light all impacting the ocean of water within you. Toxic and suppressed emotions of resentment, jealousy, shame, guilt and blame will create a toxic swamp of yuk and the more de-hydrated you are the more they flare up.

Choose your thoughts and observe each emotion with the highest level of discernment moment to moment. Water is what makes you *electro-magnetic* as water in a conductive substance as within the cerebrospinal fluid, it is mostly water. Stay hydrated for a healthy, vibrant, stress free, energised, creative, and magnetic mind. Hydrate with water, 3-4 litres a day unless your doctor has told you otherwise. It has been fascinating over the years to experiment and water is a game changer. Water is life and as a Star seed you came from the salty high vibrational waters much like the ocean and not the star dust many have been misled to be-lie-ve.

If you do not have the luxury or availability of alkaline water, bless the water you have, add salt, shake it up and stay hydrated. I have been changing the frequency of water with my hands, mind and intention of love, yes, you are more powerful than you were led to believe. This is a messenger to invite you to explore. If your emotions are toxic, then so too will the water you drink until you accept the truth of your emotions, acknowledge the messages and let them go. Hydrating with water and adding in movement will flush them out faster.

SALT

Salt is one of those vital elements that the likes of Powerade and Gatorade have manipulated the population with their clever marketing. The drinks mentioned here are high in sugar and have nothing positive or healthy for your body. You can raise the vibration of water very effectively by adding in a pinch of pink *Himalayan salt* into your bottle of water. This is not the salt such as table salt, use Himalayan, rock or sea salt.

I use a natural salt solution which is from the ocean in originality before it is created into ORMUS. It shifts the resonance of the cells and is also known an 'Elixir for the Fountain of Life.' This increases your magnetic and electrical charge and increase your mental, emotional, physical and sensual wellbeing. It is another great addiction to your natural medicine cabinet.

- Regulates the water content in the body
- Balances excess acidity from your cells, specifically brain cells

- Balances blood sugar levels
- Generates hydroelectric energy in all the cells of the body
- Reduces your ageing rate
- Regulates sleep
- Maintains *libido*
- Erectile Function – a healthy and happy hard lingam.

YOU ARE WHAT YOU EAT

The energy quality of the foods you choose to put in your mouth will impact your emotions and your energy levels. Certain foods affect the taste of sexual juices on arousal, where a women's and man's sexual juices will change. Lifestyle choices and emotions from the flesh of dead animals all impact emotions of your inner health.

The reason people eat and *crave junk food* is because their acid and alkaline balance is off. Have you ever had a big night of drinking and the next day you are hung over and crave fatty, greasy foods and more alcohol? This is because your body is acidic and when it is acidic it *craves* acidic food, yes, the sugary, trans-fatty processed foods.

Addiction cravings reduce once the internal balance is adjusted by changing the internal cellular balance to be more alkaline environment, where the drug of your choice will naturally lessen. A simple way to start to change is to munch on fresh parsley throughout the day with plenty of water hydration to assisting flush-out of unwanted toxins, old emotions and deep belly breathing. It is a sure way to get super high on greens as your body loves chlorophyl. Simple options to apply straight away.

"Truth, love and consciousness, that is what God is to me" - Ram Dass

Nature, love and consciousness provides all we need as it always has been this way. You may have been unconscious existing in fear, brainwashed and dumbed out by clever and manipulative marketing and hey, each one of YOU has been sucked in, at some point in your life!

The acid and alkaline balance of the blood and cellular health and their ability of the cells to function is key. I have tested this over many years and done many things to mess up my body, the badass that pushes the boundaries and explores the edges and live off the ledge! As you alkalise your beautiful body the more intolerance your gut will be to processed foods and anything that is removed from the natural state. Meaning when you eat them your tummy will revolt in protest and bloat. Explore what is right for your body and welcome the reactive responses in the body as a sign to listen to. The body will purge what is not aligned as it is better out than in.

- Eat foods in their most natural state as possible.
- Natural foods, meaning you can pick it from a tree and dig it up from the ground.

- Wash your fruits and vegetables in acid water to remove the toxins and then rinse in alkaline/ add bicarbonate of soda to the water, soak for 5 mins and rinse. I will be honest I am lazy with this and getting better.
- Remove toxins before eating
- Organic or locally grown as much as you can
- Support your farmers markets
- Join a community co-op for fruit and veg - it's cheap!
- Support the family farmers- not the massive corporations
- 80/20 rule – 80% whole to things you desire
- Balance is an inside job at a cellular level
- *Intuitive eating* – listen to your body as it gets easier to listen once your body is more alkaline.

- Alive or dead food- you choose?
- Meat- Ask where has it come from is it grass-fed and what are the living conditions pre-slaughter?
- Bless your food and give gratitude. Teach your children this.
- Eliminate *guilt and shame.*

The emotions that you feel whilst eating impact the energy delivery to the cells and absorption of the food via the gut. Make sure that when you eat in a restaurant you tune into the vibe of the establishment. If you have a feeling that the chef is angry, never eat the food as you will be absorbing all that toxic energy. Likewise, if you come home and your partner is bitching and complaining whilst preparing food then think twice about eating it.

I am serious; take responsibility for what you put in your mouth and the emotions you feel at the time.

Listen to your body and if you are not hungry then don't eat, it is really simple. Stay hydrated and get out in the sunshine. Eat when you are hungry and book time in each week to eat in silence. Stop forcing your children to eat when their bodies and intuition is saying otherwise, they are wiser than many adults.

ENERGY OF SUNLIGHT

One day, you and I will be taking in mostly liquid forms of nutrition and the majority of energy will come from sunlight. The more we make that evolutionary high vibration shift to a plant-based diet, the more our skin will be able to absorb the sunlight, much like a plant in '*Photosynthesis.*' I feel this is happening for many brothers and sister, scribed July 2021. Each morning set an intention to direct the energy of the sun of the skies into the central sun of your heart and then expand the auric field into your mind. This is the Sacred Ray of Freedom that can be expanded into Mother Earth, the Kingdom of life and all other human beings.

Sun creams and lotions do not stop or prevent skin cancer. Again, this *is fear-based marketing,* keeping the masses sick and maintaining the multi-billion-dollar industry of the pharmaceuticals and also the health care system. The skin needs to have exposure to sunlight and according to the National institute of health office of dietary supplements; it is healthy to have at least 20-30 minutes of naked skin exposure with no protection. Three times a week will produce enough vitamin D for the week, some may require added supplementation.

THE ROLE OF VITAMIN D

- Healthy youthful skin
- Strong bones
- Stronger teeth- less decay
- Increased energy
- Happier mood
- A healthy immunity
- Converts cholesterol to vitamin D
- Encourages the storage of ATP in the calcium deposits within the cells, vital for energy production.
- Sunlight vital to produce O2 for plants and for vegetables and fruits to be produced.

I am not a skin expert or doctor but advocate for utilising natural energy sources on our planet. I encourage you to get out in the *sun for at least 30 minutes every day.* Vitamin D deficiency is on the increase in kids and teens and maybe it is because here in Australia kids are always told to wear a sun hat and sunscreen before outdoor play, yes, even in winter! I signed a form to refuse sunscreen and my children are also very aware. The hospitals here in Australia prescribe Vitamin D to nearly all elderly patients and yet, we have the greatest sunshine here, so why is that? In India Vitamin D injections are not seen in the hospitals and this was passed on in conversation when talking to nurses in Europe and India.

Sun gazing is powerful as the sun is rising. Never look direct at the sun when it is full in the sky, have the eyelids closed if in full sunlight. Lifting your face, eyes and hands up towards the sun will increase wellbeing and calm. This simple action will allow the sun's energy to flow into your third eye, heart centre and hands.

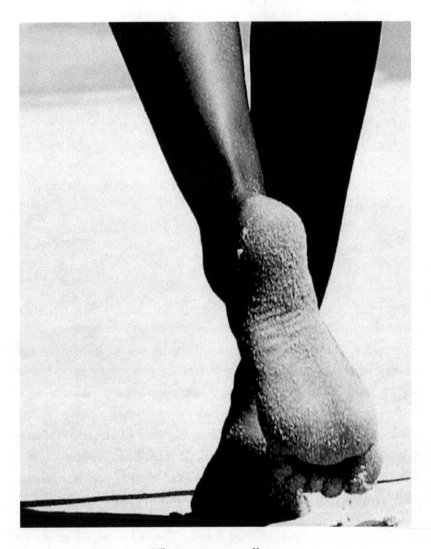

This captures it all ...

CHAPTER 6: THE MIND PRINCIPLES

"If you correct your mind, the rest will fall into place"
-Lao Tzu

MEDITATION

The mind and how the mind thinks are the Cause to what happens in your life as in the Effect, the events and experiences. You have to learn how to relax the physical body before even thinking to attempt to reach a state of awareness, known as meditation. Many are unaware as they have not been guided and are distracted by the world around and afraid to explore within. Many are 'too busy' as they are conditioned as the hamster on the wheel and chasing success. There is no way out of this, it is key to learn how to sit or lie still for 5-15 minutes with no physical movement. This first step can be the most challenging and I am not talking about sleeping.

Meditation is a state of awareness and relaxation is the phase prior to experiencing the state of meditation. The focus and concentration of the awareness is the practice. Many may never attain a state of bliss state consciousness as they have not been willing to commit to a daily practice which is consistent and steady.

Many are 'trying' many different meditation practices, and this is what I call the, *Cosmic hooker!* They never commit to anything and are open to everything. If this, is you then this is very clear of the distractions you have going on behind the scenes and a weak link in your superhuman bodysuit!

Tangibility is required as the physical body you can see and touch, meaning it is real in the manifestation of form. How can you experience the formless and have any conceptuality of it until you have begun at the more subtle level, as in form?

It is through diligent conscious awareness of the focused practice with a relaxed mind that the student begins to access the realms of the subconscious and superconscious mind. Your life is a playground of experiences, a karmic playing field of lessons and this is the true meaning of Yoga! Meditation is a life raft to accelerated change, as it creates a stable base to gain deeper inner awareness and accelerate inner transformation. A place where the individual feels safe, connected and okay with the concept of aloneness. To remember you are never alone.

The deeper the seeker transcends; the more inner wisdom that is revealed. This is where heart and mind work in harmony and symphony with one another and this opens up the ability to command ones will upon nature. You all have this ability yet most lack the discipline or will to do the inner work and the stuff no one else sees. Some key principles of information and knowledge are still hidden from public eye as the thirst to use for power or influence is a distortion when it is not used for the highest good for all humanity. Be the seeker of Self and be the pioneer of your divine path and be in integrity moment to moment to the best of your knowledge. This is not a path for everyone as they have such an attachment to their status, titles, belongings and social recognition.

A big challenge is that people have become habitually lazy, socially obedient and lacking in self-discipline and strength of will. Writing books with *this flow of creativity is a direct result of twice daily practice of meditation and booking in time for stillness.*

The practice of rigidity became a trap and even this I messed up to unravel the aspects that I was yet to see. To catch my own addiction of the bondage I was in and the love affair to the disciplined practices that created a feeling state of self-righteousness from it. To let them go and trust what naturally returned. True inner wisdom emerged in a deep inner knowing, with a playful loving lightness for life. Zoe Bell

Many have spent time in prayer, and many have shifted to incorporate the Vedic meditation into their day. Allow curious intuition to guide your way as meditation stirs creativity, evokes confidence and aligns your Soul mission and passions to access liberation. Let me be clear, nothing changes with non-action and even in stillness of meditation, movement of consciousness and action is still taking place. This is why awareness of your mindset is key to your continued Superhuman evolution.

MINDSET AWARENESS

- Indicates the frequency you are vibrating at.
- Emotions and their impact
- Projection and perception
- Perception is perception and not reality.

- Reality is Truth which is love/Consciousness
- Cause V Effect
- Discern what is real and what is an illusion?
- *'Rebellious Defiance'* to follow your hearts passion.

You experience different states of consciousness during your daily lives, sleep, full alertness, half asleep, and daydreaming. This frequency is measured by scientist's EEG. This creates a sound creates a vibration at a deep level. A life raft to change and deep transformation. All feelings and emotions create a sound vibration. Are you beginning to see the connections? Let us explore the brains frequency of electrical energy and how it changes depending on your state of awareness?

The Different States

- GAMMA- Highly alert and conscious – 30-80 HZ – Healing with Tibetan singing bowls – Tone of G - Binaural beats.

- BETA – full alert mode 15-30HZ- Conscious to the outside world

- ALPHA- daydreaming 9-14 Hz – adult beginners of meditation can reach.

- THETA- a waking dream 4-8Hz – no thought – experienced practitioners of meditation reach this state – transcendence and deep restoration.

- DELTA- deep sleep 1-3Hz- where the physical body heals and comes back into balance- Dreamless sleep.

Frequency and Vibration

Nothing rests. Everything moves. Everything vibrates.

At the most fundamental level, the Universe and everything which compromises it is *pure vibratory energy manifesting itself* in different ways. The Universe has no 'solidity', as such. *Matter* is merely *energy* in a state of vibration.

Natural Law seminar with Mark Passio

Cause and Effect

- Cause – Intention creates thoughts and emotions.
- Effect - What happens and the experiences, the action, reactions and resulting manifestation of fear or Love

Cause and effect are one of the Key principles in Natural Law.

Every Cause has its Effect and every Effect has its Cause. Everything happens according to law Chance is but a name for Law not recognized. There are many planes of causation, but nothing escapes the Law.

There are manifested realities that have formed due to their underlying causes. The plane of effects constitutes that which has already occurred. As such, no power to affect change lies here, because that which has already occurred cannot un-occur, it has become That Which is (Truth). Human consciousness seems to be trapped upon the Plane of Effects, meaning that humanity, as a whole remains *ignorant of the underlying causes* which they themselves set into motion and which led to self-inflicted suffering in their lives. – *Natural Law seminar, Mark Passio*

THE PINEAL GLAND

The Pineal Gland is a pinecone shaped structure that once awakened is often misunderstood as others may want to sleep with you. This energy is powerful and can be manipulative when used for gaining sexual pleasure, this is something to be aware of. Always take responsibility for your choices and be discerning when you access this potency, as it is pure light awareness. As your inner glow increases more people are magnetically drawn to you so be the reflection of love that holds them in the highest of respect. This is healing energy and yes, it is sensual in nature.

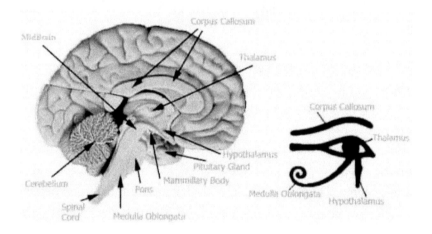

To See beyond the Eyes of Judgment and See through the Sacred Heart and the Masculine EYE and the Feminine EYE.

The Egyptians were aligned with inner seeing and inner knowing. Their heads were shaped differently as they had enlarged pineal glands. The Egyptian's were ET, you only have to research how tall they were. We are remembering to access realms covered up and hidden over many years.

There is a little doorway at the base of the skull, which I refer to as the God

Spot. This is also called the 'The 'Mouth of God' and the 'Golden Chalice', anatomically known as the *Medulla Oblongata.*

I discovered a door near the Cerebellum near the Medulla Oblongata and had the clearest of visions. As if I was remote viewing, as if watching a movie. Perhaps it was the Medulla Oblongata, there are many doors to explore! The path reveals when you least expect the seeing.

Keep exploring the sacred chambers and be curious as the Golden child explores. Notice shifts in the body on rising, like natural cracking as in adjustments of the C1-C2 joint in the neck. A simple nodding upon waking, chin to chest whilst lying flat in bed is assisting a natural adjustment.

This doorway to consciousness to reveal clear seeing and messages to be delivered at God speed. This little doorway has been blocked for many years and is now opening. Once it is opened, it remains open.

This opening will activate the *Arc of Covenant* making your access to Universal intelligence far greater than it has done so far and a doorway to Cosmic energy. This activation aligns the human with the *Avatar Self* and the light body becomes the main transmitter. The alignment with the false power of the patriarchal system, can thus no longer exist in the individual.

Other key aspects

- The Corpus Callosum, is the *Sacred Bridge* of the brain Hemispheres. Do you remember this is strengthened through the practice of contemplation?

- To explore the *Garden of Eden* is the cross the rainbow bridge and through a door to the right and into the *infinite realm of imagination.*
- *Heaven on Earth* is accessed through the sacred heart that Shines light upon the Mouth of God, the projection is viewed by light shining upon the pituitary and viewed by the Pineal gland.

Tips for opening Your inner seeing and Insight

- Fluoride in the tap water creates cloudy insight and foggy thinking. It dumbs us down and creates calcification around the pineal gland so that it does not function the way it is designed. Change your water and your toothpaste.
- Drink tulsi tea – to assist.
- Watching the news - clouds vision - Give it a try! Turn it off.
- Dark chocolate assist to decalcify the pineal and for fun add strawberries and berries as I've been told and experimented with this yummy mix, this boosts the goodness in the dark chocolate- as Vitamin C
- Meditation will assist to produce DMT naturally. yes, you get high on life.
- I get high with breathing practices - you have a natural pharmacy of the drugs you need, and many are hibernating in your brain.

Life is a journey…

- Exploring is your human right
- Curiosity is required

- This is a map and compass to guide
- You must do the practices
- To get out of your head
- Healing and awakening - a journey.
- The passion for learning - a limitless gift

Vedic meditation practice awakens...

- Frequency and control of thoughts
- Healing and psychic abilities
- Sensual power and prowess
- Confidence & sexual magnetism
- Self-esteem & self-worth
- The pineal gland to secrete DMT naturally

- Younger glow and lightness in being
- Creativity & self-expression – to write many books!
- An ability to shift beyond attachment
- Acceptance and excitement of change
- Feeling Joy and fearlessly leaping into the unknown.

Leading to...

- Stronger, deeper connection to all that is
- The power of the subconscious and supraconscious mind

- Deeper spiritual connection with self
- Ability to listen and trust gut instincts
- Increased focus and ability to sustain pleasure
- Knowing you are deserving

- Confidence in body image
- Improved self-esteem
- Stronger, more creative imagination for fantasies.
- Calmer and more centered.

Yoga is life and meditation a life raft to trust in the external changing landscape. This is a key to unify, harmonise and bring inner *balance and peace* for the individual and into the collective ocean of consciousness.

Meditation for some may be *walking in nature,* dancing to music, moving the body, singing, driving a sports car as it was created, and it can be anything that accesses joy within. Be present moment to moment as you feel into your multidimensional selves. Find what it is for you and make time for a consistent practice every day! There is no one size fits all; it's your adventure and your journey. I share my own and there are many paths and ways up the mountain.

BREATHING

Expanding on Universal magnetism, breathing is essential to become present with the moment and You can breathe your way into happiness, sensual magnetism and vibrant wellbeing. Breathing connects you directly with the environment as a direct path of consciousness and the breath is life.

Many unaware people and those running fear programs take breathing for granted as they simply are not aware, until they are made aware. Anxiety is a message to breathe OUT and let go of the worrying /panic of the future and a message to become aware!

A clear sign is to address habitual wrong thinking, irrational emotions/fears and not being present in the now. For years of guiding others how to breathe, direct and simply to follow guidance is required. Many are *unconsciously incompetent* at first before being taught how to re-learn how to breathe. As young kids you knew how to breathe before the faulty wiring of the mind-body programs of fear reactivity.

The sacred rivers within and the spine is the structure for the breath to flow. To climb your way up Jacob's ladder, beyond the matrix and out of the sand pit of the noise of unconscious living.

- **Ida** - Feminine - the Mother
- **Pingala** - Masculine - The Father
- **Shushumna - The Central channel** - Middle Way of the Rising

The masculine and the feminine and upon this path called life we are learning to navigate the natural push- pull of the nature, within and without. The dance is to become effortless and access the *'middle way'* in all ways and within all directions of the winds.

This is how the 3 rivers move and communicate.

You each are here to master your own nervous and electromagnetic energy systems by taking self-responsibility of the inner work. To be the change and share the high frequency of love, light, peace, harmony and abundance for all upon the Earths grid.

Make a commitment to you to each day spend five minutes being grateful for your breath and marvel in what a gift it is to breathe. Simply, observe the breath without fixing or changing it, become aware of the air moving in and the air moving out. Rewind back to 'Wildflower' and all the breathing practices.

Breathing to balance - *Nadi Shodhana – Here is a refresher of Alternate nostril breathing.* A path to balance the masculine and feminine energetic currents restoring inner harmony.

- Sit upright in a comfortable seat.
- Either on the floor, on a chair or against the wall.
- Legs crossed or out straight
- Relax your shoulders and body

- Using your right hand, rest your first two fingers, lightly touching the space between your eyebrows
- This is the area of the 3rd eye
- Your thumb is resting on the outside of your right nostril
- Your 4th and 5th finger lightly resting against the left nostril
- Gaze to the tip of your nose and softly close your eyes
- Tip of the tongue resting on the top of the plate just behind the front top teeth
- Allow your breath to move freely in and out of the nostril
- Make a mental note which nostril is more open!
- Take a deep breath in and block off the right nostril
- Exhale out the left
- Inhale through the left
- Block off the left
- Exhale right
- Inhale right
- Block off right
- Exhale left
- Keep rotating in this manner
- Ensuring no force yet full emptying of the lungs.
- Two – five minutes
- Finish the round by exhaling through the left nostril.

Breathing Practices to explore

- *Breathing to revitalise the mind-* Short and fast inhales through the nose- over-oxygenation – short bursts.

- *Sexual arousal for a man* - Opening up the right nostril, so the right nostril flow is more open. Block off the left nostril- breathe in and out of the right nostril – for 5 minutes before sensual activity and intimate connection.

- *Sexual arousal for a woman* - Opening up the left nostril, so flow is more open through the left. Block off the right nostril and breathe in and out of the left nostril – 5 minutes before sensual activity and intimate connection.

- *Breathing for magnetism, manifestation and attraction*- alternate nostril breathing and Vedic meditation which I can teach you, this is a process that is for the advanced student.

- *Breathing for deep and lasting orgasms*- This is taught one on one. This is explored in Chapter 9, in the section on the Mer-Ka-Ba. This is an advanced technique that needs one on one attention from a teacher. Begin with breathing practices and some form of meditation as this will bring deeper awareness to the body.

Like everything, consistency is key to having a discipline to strengthen at the foundational level. Simplicity to complexity and being gentle with the Nervous system so it has time to adapt and change and to then return to basics as higher frequency comes into the vessel to be assimilated and navigated. The nervous system is to be respected beyond what the ego wants! If you force it, you will get served onto your ass as you cannot push against of change Natural Law.

- *Breathing into Oneness – 'Sensual Sacred Unity'*

Sit opposite your partner and begin to synch your breath with one another as you dive deep into one another's eyes and feel into their breath. While you are sitting there, you will be sharing the same ether, the energy around one another and within one another. This is potent and such a beautiful experience and one that we need to do more of.

- *Breathing into Oneness- a 'Remote Love Union'*

Sit as if you can feel one another's blueprint in front of you. Begin to feel into the energetic waves as you both empty your minds and where hearts become one as the unified breath moves in and out. This is an advanced practice, and a deep sensual experience can be explored when both and meeting in unconditional love. The energy has shifted beyond sexual and a powerful sensual force of nature and meeting in higher dimensions of consciousness.

This is where you start to have an experience of Oneness and the barriers of perception dissolved, to see yourself in the other and them in you, as you are one. This also goes with kissing, your mouths and breathes in synch, a poetic potion of passion drawing you closer into one another, a sweet wave of inner bliss and ecstasy. Like everything, always discern what feels peaceful and what feels persistent. Energy that is persistent and pushy is a red flag warning so use your discernment that is strengthening with courageous action.

EMOTIONS

Emotions impact your energetic frequency. Begin to have awareness to the shifting tides of your emotions as the ever-changing ocean as emotions are messages from Spirit. The Spirit body that is within your bodysuit. The key is to invite curiosity with zero judgment. Be the observer in a zoomed-out viewing with loving awareness. Notice your emotions and see them with honour and gratitude to support each release. The path to ease and grace is to allow them to be seen, felt and then allowing them to pass through you within a space of stillness.

I hope that by now you are seeing that your story and divine journey are perfect for what you are here to learn and explore. Choose your thoughts, emotions and feeling state and if you don't like what you are thinking, bring it into the light to accept the thought. Ask what it is showing you about yourself? Acknowledge it and explore what it is revealing on a deeper level, then when ready, let it go. Learn to embrace change as everything is changing and emotions so too shall pass. Be fearless in expressing your emotions and be aware where you lash out at others, own your reactions, show redemption and forgive yourself. Know that each time you acknowledge the emotion by calling it out you are freeing yourself and growing into expanded states of consciousness. It is a wild ride, and you will all make it. Hold an inner state of gratitude as this internal shift will bringing a sense of wellbeing and rewire at the causal level. Infuse small offerings of gratitude into your life every day, like fresh air, clean water, play and choose to be around those who love you. Start small and set goals to aim for whilst practicing gratitude every day.

When emotions are unexpressed and suppressed this translates to dying slowly on the inside. It is a cause for depression, apathy and giving up on You!

CHAPTER 7: THE SPIRIT PRINCIPLES

"When you do things from your Soul, you feel a river moving in you"

-Rumi

NATURE

Nature holds the key to all that you need. This is about connecting to all that lights up and ignites your Free Spirit that came here to play, explore being human and to know what love is. Mother Earths hand holds you within your most fragile of times. She is limitless and resilient, and SHE is within each and every one of you. Getting into nature with the Earth beneath your feet is one of the greatest ways to access Spirit and soothe your warrior heart and re-claim the child innocence. Nature is a place to come back into your natural state of balance and find your inner harmony as nature holds a key to awakening the remembrance of Your Souls medicine. Escape the urban jungle with those you love and retreat into the wildness of nature and reconnect to Spirit. Kick off our shoes as much as possible and walk around barefoot. Climb trees, hug them, touch rocks, the Earth and be open to the Great Mother and the Father Sky and Sun of Spirits wisdom. Think about how you feel after being in nature, at the beach with salty skin and wild hair, cleansing away from the noisy city.

You will feel better for getting back to your roots, within nature and living off the land. It is time to align with your free Spirit and the Moon. Get swinging in trees, awaken your inner child, unleash your playful spirit and set your Soul on fire!

Your 10 toes caress the flesh of Mother Gaia as you walk upon her flesh. To breathe through your feet as a conduit between what is above and that which is below. Your 5 toes represent, *Peace, Love, Harmony, Unity and Freedom.* Walk with intention and be a powerful conduit of these Free-Queen-sees. Your feet have Star portal points/ Chakras within them and the Earth Star of the Star constellation Pisces beneath your feet, and it is time to dance upon the Earth.

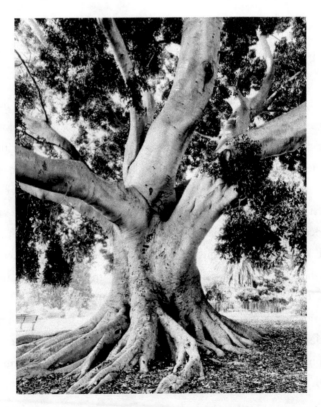

CONNECT IN NATURE

- Take off your shoes and go barefoot.
- Explore new places in nature with your family
- Dance upon the Earth as your ancestors did.
- Place your hands on a tree trunk and see if the tree speaks to you. You may feel a humming in your hands, a sweet vibration and warm glow within your heart, the ancient ones speak to me in this way.
- Get your hands in the dirt, plant some flowers or herbs and take care of them every day and guide your children.
- Get to the ocean, watch, listen and play within the waves.
- Feel the sand between your toes
- Get dirty in the mud and even get naked in the mud
- Yoga on the beach and the Earth
- Immerse into the natural salt water
- Immerse into the cold mountain stream
- Watch the sunrise and sunset
- Jump in puddles and care not for getting wet
- Paint one another with mud and dirt- it's fun
- Be painted naked and pained in natures landscape
- Sunbathe naked in the wildness of nature
- Go for walks in the mountains and bushlands
- Go camping and rough it in a swag
- Sleep under the moon and stars
- Go make-up free and feel the sunlight upon your bare skin

- Support causes that are for restoring and preserving the planet
- Remember your mission on Earth.

EVOKE YOUR PASSIONS

Your passions are connected to your Spirits liberation. You naturally light up with rich raw emotions that over-spill like liquid gold when connecting to your passions. This is the nitro within the magnetic energy and a Key to tapping into limitless creativity whilst having an insatiable zest for living life. Choose to create a fresh and inspired habit of booking time-in for you each and every day to immerse into your passions. Your life is valuable and connecting to your passions is an act of self-love. You have to make it happen by being responsible for your choices and how you spend or waste your time. Nothing shifts until you shift.

Put on your own oxygen mask, before putting on others oxygen mask.

It is your passion that gives you to energy to jump out of bed excited about your day and is super inspiring to be around.

- Are you living your passions?
- Do you know what makes your heart and soul sing?
- Do you do something every day you feel passionate about?
- This is a Key to your heart-soul path.
- Start to book time in *at least* for five- minutes every day.
- Be supportive and adore your partner's passion and purpose!

Check-in with your partner to see if he or she is making time in for their passions. Many men forget about themselves and are placing everyone else before them. This is unhealthy!

Encourage your children and be the example by connecting to your passions as actions speak louder than words. Create creative space with less rules as their inner guidance will lead the way. Children intuitively know, so as a parent be mindful not to interrupt their deep connection in play. There is a direct connection to the *sensual inner power* generated from connecting with passions. Creative souls are more sensual and passionate about life. Begin to be less controlling and see what shifts in all areas your life.

- Are you living a life of freedom?
- Or playing the victim of self-imprisonment?
- You get to choose, so what is it?
- You have one shot at this lifetime, are you truly living it?

Once your passion is unleashed there is a *fire in your belly* that is relentless and will assist to tap into a resource of unlimited energy and vitality. When this awakens you chip away at your vision and dreams until you create the vision, and no matter how many times you fall, you will continue to get up and start all over again. Your deepest passions are a reflection of your Soul purpose and your compass to why you are here on Earth. This is how some can work for 16 hours straight and keep going until it is done, yes, beautiful passionate people who are stepping up and making it happen!

ADVENTURE & PLAY

Plan adventures with your friend's, partner and family and be less serious and enjoy life. This does not have to cost money and many times the best times are spontaneous and all about the people that are there. It is all about the company and the collective vibe that are present within the moment. It is the collective energy that makes it magical, be it a small and intimate group of a larger group of Souls.

There is something beautiful about watching two people lovingly act silly together, behaving as those no one else existed. - Steve Maraboli

Book a trip by yourself, get out of your comfort zone and explore new places as you never know whom you may meet. Explore fantasies in your mind and share your deepest thoughts, dreams and desires with your intimate partner. Your mind is a safe place to explore, and you get to invite in whom you like. These are your thoughts and unless you explore with your mind something new, you will never know. Stay open to exploring with your curiosity within the world of fantasy and imagination and see where it takes you, they are your secret thoughts, so enjoy them.

Those that are unable to be silly will never have 'Peak experiences of all consuming states of immense love, joy and happiness'. They are locked into the robotic rat race of the walking dead.

The greatest adventure you can have is doing something different and following through on a feeling, listing to the spirit guides and trusting in divine timing. Life can be as fun as you choose to make it! I see my life and all lives as one big adventure and you can see it however you choose to see it, moment to moment as the changing landscape of your life. Perhaps, begin to explore a lighter view on life and see what happens.

Rewind back to your childhood as that is the perfect place to start and a key to your sparkly aspects.

- What did you love to do as a child?
- What adventures make your heart sing?
- What is holding you back from exploring new places?
- Do you find fun in even the most mundane exercises?
- Can you find a way to have fun every day?
- If time and money were not an issue, what would you do?
- Where would you travel?

See these as seeds to inspire you to awaken your curiosity in each and every moment you get to experience this magical adventure called life.

SELF-GROWTH

It is vital to cultivate the willingness and discipline to keep doing those things to feel good and also address the things that trigger You. Make no excuses when taking responsibility for your wellbeing and the way you show up in the world, moment to moment. This is a vital step to becoming the best version of yourself as you continue to grow and evolve. The learning never ends! Once you go down the rabbit hole of truth there is no going back and yet many stay stuck, as they are addicted to the programs of limitation playing out. Many enjoy feeling bad, the bullshit victim story and living in pain. Each are creating it all by allowing their circumstances of the past to define this now. It takes courage to be persistent as it never about the destination and wow, is it a colourful path and never dull. Some are addicted to being stuck as they have a deep fear of failure, and this is where procrastination kicks in. Self-growth is a part of your Spiritual evolution and may feel easy to start, and then you don't want to go any further down the rabbit hole of the unknown. Many are placing exploring the healing and pushing the pause button as they are scared and know that space of required to go deep. The sad part is they are caught up in the flashy aspects of success and will use excuses of it's not the right time. Life is beautiful and will assist to rebalance where there is no other option that to explore the inner healing. Never be afraid to take a few steps, you are worth it and the leaps beyond cannot be described.

Be aware if you have become the 'self-help junkie' that is constantly dissecting your life and never coming up for air to celebrate living. Even shadow work has become a badge of honour for some, and this is a ploy of the clever ego.

All to seek attention for the wounds and the unhealed trauma, to feed the insecurity that is drowning within. No matter where you are at is exactly where you are meant to be. It is the things that you do each day that will reap the rewards, and not just when you feel like it, or suddenly need it. It is a lifestyle adjustment to knowing thy self.

- *Read a book for 5 minutes* in the morning after your meditation, at lunch and before bed. A powerful technique to implement whilst standing.
- *Listen to uplifting speakers* that inspire you to take action and evoke a desire in your belly.
- *Listen to topics you are passionate* about and begin to turn off the news.
- Go to sleep with a book *under my pillow* to absorb information and knowledge as you sleep and then begin to integrate.
- *Sleep listening to audio,* as your sub-conscious absorbs.
- *Keep a journal* and write to get it out, no care for grammar and write with intentional mind dumping.
- Keep notes and place them around the house, *quotes and statements* that mean something to you now and even more powerful, the essence you wish to be more like.
- Write and live your passions as much as possible.
- Go to events that inspire you or be in your own space.
- Study those and follow those who inspire you.
- Be mindful who and what you listen to.
- Tell yourself how awesome you are, every day and whatever you do, *never give up!*

- Be present and the best you can be with those you love.
- Book You time in everyday as a top priority.
- Be uniquely you and care fewer what others think.
- Mediate everyday- it has the potential to unlock your inner wisdom! 20 min x 2/day. Find a meditation that works for you and can be a consistent aspect to your living.

CONNECTION WITH OTHERS

Connect with like-minded people, this may mean having a clear up of your friends and then making space for a *fresh lit and light crew*. This may sound a bit drastic for some; it's all your choice. I absolutely love having a cull of the list as it is like spring cleaning your wardrobe. If you haven't worn it and it still has the tags on it, then maybe it is not meant to be there. There are those pieces that you will always have, this is like people in your life. The friends you thought you have, maybe willing to stab you in the back at the first opportunity they have. In an attempt to trample on you, so they look better, be grateful when these people show their true colours as you can then cut them out of your life.

The truth prevails and will always come out and those that are evolved and awake will see the truth, which is Love. See each ending as a fresh beginning and unless you clear up and clear up the Karmic vibration, the same smell and lesson will return.

Align with those that challenge growth and you can have rich conversations with beyond an alienation of opposing views, hold compassion for all. Reminder, that the five people you share your time with are who you will become like. This is about becoming your own Guru and never giving our power away again in some hierarchy or system of order. You are all learning, and you will all graduate, and it will be a matter of timing. You have a choice to evolve and leap or to manifest the unwanted and everything you require clearing in the 3rd physical density.

Share your passions to connect through dance, voice, music and touch. Find a group or a cause you are passionate about and be willing to stand for something to make the World a better place for all. Connection may be sharing your wisdom with others via social media as in content creation. I feel people are craving one-to-one connection and there is a shift within supporting at a local community level. Connection is evolving beyond the senses and into the intuitive higher vibrational communication of Soul families and this is where you begin to expand ways in which you communicate and connect beyond locality or convenience.

I discover the deepest connections with Spirit are within silence, as I am already home. You are whole, you never were broken, and Your life is a gift so don't waste it by non-action and being lazy in old excuses. There are many un-purposeful humans that have lost their will to do anything with their life.

Connection with self is vital as if you cannot spend time with yourself then why would anyone else want to? It is beautiful to *love your own company*. I absolutely love those first connections with another you feel drawn to, a side-ways glance, a smile with no attachment, to be in that state of feeling good, free and unlimited possibility.

The coffee shop chats are rich as you never know whom you will meet and what the Universe has in store for you. Enjoy each interaction in presence as the connection may lift the other up in more ways than you realise at the time. Ways in which people connect.

- Groups
- Tribes
- Community
- Social media
- The Path of the Lone Wolf (this is me)
- One to one in intimacy

Whether it is connecting in small groups or one to one, dive in deep and be free with no competition for space to be heard. I love being with myself, in quiet or listening to music and drums in the background. Be one of those people who goes out and shares the feeling of rich passion, joy and love, share your shine with the world. If the energy is not to your liking, then leave quietly. Now you see me, now you don't, you get the picture.

I love to be taken to my edge, to feel challenged and to free fall forwards into a fresh adventure. I choose my space wisely and selectively and will step away to always attend to my heart to honour my Spirit. Learn to listen to others with your entire being and be present enough to witness everything they are saying.

Your vibe will attract your Tribe; you don't like your tribe, then cultivate a different vibe! A lone wolf will walk alone as other lone wolfs will find You! The Ones that have stepped away from the socialized hive mind.

There may come a time where your tribe gets smaller and smaller, this can un-settle some, for me this is *bliss*. It is a place of contentment to depending less on others, to hold those dearest in your heart, possibly all scattered across the globe and each one of them living their Soul truth and remembering your Galactic Soul Family.

Being of Service

It is your purpose to share your gift with the world and vital for the evolution of the human species beyond the depopulation agenda and a world of asexual Zombies. Once your passion and purpose are realised then any inaction of sharing it will become increasingly uncomfortable. You are doing your Free Spirits Soul mission and humanity a dis-service. The path of service to others is one of devotion and will present many challenges to test resilience, readiness and in this much self-sacrifice. It is a path to be walked alone and initiation in the wilderness is key.

To serve can begin with something you share with your family and friends and your gifts are coming from your heart. If the head is leading, then this is about 'self.' To serve from the heart, is to be a vessel for source to flow through. Start local as this is not about fame or fortune.

This is about sharing your unique gifts with the world and most importantly your family. This will have a positive impact in all your relationships and also your energy levels. Any situation you can flip into a positive and leave a positive impression wherever you go and to give without the expectation to receive anything in return.

The best anyone can do, is to make use of the gifts they have been given and sharing them with the world. You each have unique gifts, now it is time to express them and be free.

- People will remember the impact that you had on them and not the things you do, it is all about being present with them.

- Give your children and those you love your presence and not presents! Guide you children by your example to give to those who may have fewer opportunities, a friend in need and see the best in all.

- Give people your time and presence and know your value on your time. Never under sell yourself; this all comes down to self-love and self-worth and this inner standing is beyond money exchange.

- Never under value, power and warmth of a smile, it is free and says a million words. Make the world a brighter place and light up the world with your smile.

- This is not about telling others who you think you are, allow them to see who you are by your being-ness of you and not some flashy title.

The beautiful love affair between the Trinity of Mind, Body and Spirit to access the child like innocence by aligning with Natural and Spiritual Law. These are rituals and are vital to truly understand how the Mer-Ka-Ba integrates into your existence- Explored in chapter 9.

In each moment you have a conscious choice in who you show up as and how you choose to express. As you integrated the mind-body and spirit practices there will be less over-thinking of the mind as you are beginning to master your thoughts and allow your sense of wonder and imagination to be free. You are more aware of the distraction and there is less attachment to the background chatter.

Invite more play, dance and imagination into your day - Z

Be discerning in all your choices and applied actions which translates to applying wisdom (integrated knowledge) and honouring intuition in the matrix game. Methods and Principles teach discipline to assist with the foundations of the structure; they instill focus and a strong will to stay on track. Keep bringing the entity of you back to you and see each practice as fun and not a chore. Your individual journey takes persistence and yes you will go off track, it is human behaviour as we are habitual by nature. The smarter and more you adapt the more efficiently you will get back on track until you catch the ego in the driving seat of entitlement. Always look forward to connecting to the things that cultivate a sense of wellbeing and give a sense of feeling good as a sensual soul. As the inner will of the human strengthens and intentions purify into clarity, the Spirit becomes free in each and every moment. A renewed sense of inner peace and calmness surrounding you, as when you become still, the peace and joy finds you.

Be willing to align with The Mind-Body-Spirit Principles with the pure intention is to radiate Unconditional Love.

It is time to remember how to restore inner and outer peace and radiance so you too can be a clear conduit for a higher resonance of light to flow through. It is your mission to activate your specific codes, commit to growth and play a key role in Hu-man evolution.

Welcome home to your heart's vocabulary of restoring innocence of the inner child which is your Free Spirit and badass emergence as Soul! The rising of the golden child from the divine union of the masculine and feminine forces within and rising as the middle way.

CHAPTER 8: RELEASE THE ENERGETIC BLOCKS

"Take Care of your Body. It is the only place You have to live in"

- Jim Rohn

MARINATING THE MEAT BODYSUIT

It is yoga play time and exploration into how you can work with specific yoga postures to engage a deeper translation between the 7-Star Portals / Chakras in your bodysuit and the cosmos. A guide to assist integration of movement, breath and sound and the emotionality that can release and be processed by each energy portal. Below is some Yoga play in the hood

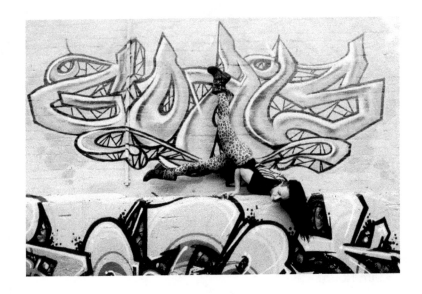

No matter your yoga experience I have made this, so it is available to all levels.

With all these following yoga postures the key is to hold the posture and breathe calmly in and out through the nose for three to five minutes. If exhaling out of the mouth feels more available, do that as long as you are not mouth breathing which will drain your energy. You can always begin with a breath count of in for 3 and out for 3 for 1-minute in and out of the nose and then progress.

Ways to Wake up Your Spine Daily.

- Forward fold
- Modified forward fold

- Forward fold in bed
- Find a playground, hang from the monkey bars.

To be your loving guide it is vital to explain something that can and may happen as you explore the yoga journey. Yoga postures, movements and the breath all work with the nervous system to assist a connection with your emotional body. When combined they will stir up stuck, old emotions as they are beginning to find a way to release. It is key to mention this in case you find yourself in fear reactivity and go into panic, and then you avoid future yoga practice out of fear. Fear reactivity is very real and is a doorway for healing and it is not about going into the story of the emotion either.

FEAR REACTIVITY

This is where the stress response becomes so great that you become immobilised by fear. This I have experienced first-hand more than three times personally when releasing the physical blocks of tension and old trauma from the tissues. I recall it kicking in 30 mins after a yoga class at the beginning of my yoga journey in 2004 and I was overcome with panic and froze in a car park, I called my teacher and he guided me as I thought I was going crazy. What is being stirred up are old responses of reaction and resistance wired into the nervous system. As it kicked in, I became frozen in fear, and this is what is known as a fear reactivity response. I have had many clients have this happen and loving guidance is required.

In the moment of fear reactivity, you will want to run, escape in panic and the key is to remain presence in stillness. The less you move the better, trust, be still and breathe through and into the reactivity. Yes, breathe into the reaction. It will pass and like anything and everything, it is all waves of energy to be experienced as the present witness. Nothing ever stays the same. If you avoid going into what you resist and avoid then it will get louder and over time more blocks of resistance are created in the density of the body. The choices are to evolve or become denser.

Reminder: *Pain is a wise messenger to move & invite in the fear*

Many are stuck in survival mode on a daily basis, caught within the fear game by what they hear, watch, read and the daily self-destructive thought patterns. This survival mentality leads to the need and desire to have power and manipulate and dominate others. I see this in those that hide behind titles of self-importance and the ego driven success game and all I see are weak people. Codependency is a form of inflexibility and a resistance to walk alone and do the inner work on self.

Learn to get your hands and knees dirty, do the inner work to adapt and evolve.

Your physical, mental and emotional bodies are vehicles to living a life of inner freedom. The mind is powerful with a wild imagination yet, with a stubborn 'over-thinking' computer. To strengthen 'will' you have to activate it through disciplines, and practices. This then gives greater access to all aspects of the mind. You have to teachable and willing to meet the pain and your fear and emotions at the door and invite them in by exploring the resistance within the physical body.

You service, love and care for your car and yet, how much daily loving attention and investment do you give to your mind-body vessel? Your answer will shift and change over time and taking the first step is always the hardest, you have to begin with acceptance to where you are at! Many are so attached to their 4-wheel vehicles or motorbikes yet treat the 2-legged mind-bodysuit like shit. They bitch and complain, placing guilt, shame and blame on others and this leads to sickness or an injury.

Illness is a state of mind that manifests in the body to wake you up from the deep sleep.

Supported Crow – Bakasana

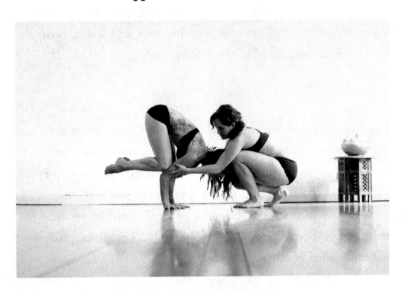

Bakasana, also known as crow, is a great posture to face your fears of falling as it may evoke fear reactivity to assist transformation. With loving guidance, directed support and confidence in the individual magic happens. Soon the limiting belief shifts into an empowered experience of flying. With the right guidance, if you have arms, you can do this, yes, even after shoulder issues, it is all about balance and has a strong core activation. The hands are working to ground, and the centre of gravity shifts to find the sweet pivot spot. The feeling of going too far is the sweet spot of finding balance. Give this a go when you feel ready to explore facing your fear of falling, look out in front as when look directly down this is where your attention and body will go!! Get to a yoga class or book in for some yoga play and learn how to fly and I can guide anybody no matter where you live.

Much of humanity exists in a state of learnt helplessness and we the light warriors are here to walk you home and to guide you how to leap and fly!

WHAT IS THE AMYGDALA HIJACK?

The Amygdala hijack mentioned in *Breaking Free* is an immediate and overwhelming emotional response out of proportion to the stimulus, as it has triggered a more significant threat. The amygdala is the part of the brain that handles emotions. When this "Amygdala Hijack' happens, it shuts down the neo-cortex, the *thinking brain* and this is the part of the rational brain. The message that is communicated with the amygdala is a run, flight or freeze situation.

This can lead to you reacting irrationality and destructively. Learning to change this reaction is for the individual to start implementing changes in order to learn self-control. Many who have been experienced trauma and experienced similar 'trigger' situations, the reaction gets layered upon one another. Meaning the reaction gets stored in your emotional memory bank. This part of the brain is called the Limbic System. This can lead to reactions without any logic or reason, causing your body to go into a run, fight or freeze response.

I was stuck within this and as triggers now arise with awareness you can shift it. The key is having the discipline to see each reaction when it presents and then re-wiring the nervous system with an upgraded and calm response. The child's pose yoga posture is a great tool and safe place to start from. Feeling out of control is scary and not a fun place to be living within 24/7. My advice is that right in the moment of the reaction find a safe place to come into child's pose, stop all talking and drop into the posture, rest your forehead on the floor or your hands, be still and breathe.

By constantly reacting, you are blocking your flow of life and looping the chaotic mess upon your path of self-destruct, dropping to the floor is a great place to land and to begin to change your life, from the ground up.

Childs Pose

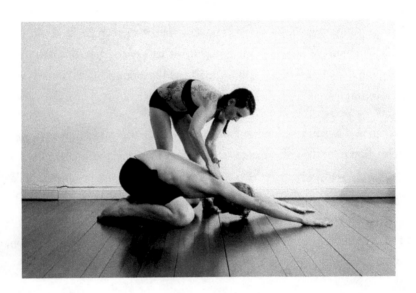

Some wise words of advice, if you are going to explore the partner child's pose, before you touch another in this position, always ask permission before assisting. They may punch you if they feel threatened. You cannot know what is happening on the inside and giving space is such a gift and the nervous system in reaction requires space to breathe. Assisting to release trauma is not something you jump into it is process that requires guidance and learning about the phases of trauma in your study of seeking knowledge and then through integration of your own inner healing. If you receive a yes, then explore this posture and be mindful of size differences and take it slow. The one on the base controls the posture so communicate using your words as there is no force required. Once in position breath in synch with one another as the added weight invites a deeper opening and offering for a supported emotional release.

This is beautiful to do with your partner when naked and to breathe into one another. Feel the magic un-folding and the delicious skin to skin contact as your bodysuits communicate beyond words.

If you find getting your bottom to your heels in child's pose challenging, place a pillow behind your knees. If the tops of our feet are restricted and you feel discomfort, then this is a great posture for you.

Assisted Childs Pose

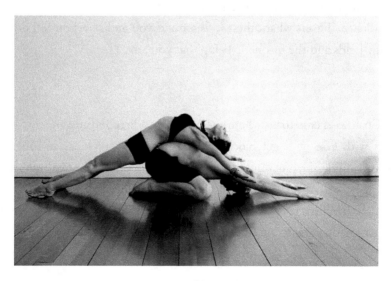

THE ENERGY WHEEL SYSTEM

Now to explore these energy portals within the body that mimic wheels spinning really fast and are often called *Chakras*. For many, they are blocked or leaking vital energy due unawareness of how to work with them and past life experiences of physical, emotional and psychological trauma which impacted the specific aspects of healthy human development. These energy wheels make up the energetic body and they have the ability to deliver messages to You and to others and they are powerful portals for clearing old blocks. By addressing these dense and often stagnant blocks of energy, flow can be restored into fluidity. As you evolve your body vessel will have a greater ability and capacity to hold and embody more light.

As mentioned earlier energy is constantly moving up and down, left to right, right to left, round and round, in and out of your bodysuit. This life-force energy moves in beautiful cyclical patterns all of which are rays of radiant light. This is how the auric field is created which is rainbow light in radiance. This is what others feels around you and how you feel others energy fields and the magnetic being that you are.

See Chakras as crossroads where energy changes direction and energy either flows with ease or it get blocked from emotional, physical and mental obstructions at the junctions. There are over 100 chakras in our body, and 13 Chakras of the 13 Star constellations/Star Portals. I will guide you through the first seven chakras as these are most relevant to what is happening on a conscious and evolutionary level for humanity. There are 72,000 Nadis, where omnipresent life-force energy flows with the 3 main

Nadi's energy channels in the body, Ida, Pingala and Sushumna.

Blockages represent different areas of the body and are related to your human development through childhood and into adulthood. Reflect back to *the Womb healing in Wildflower* as I go through the development of each chakra in each 7-year cycles. This is how you learnt through survival as a species. Try to understand that they are swirls of spinning energy with stagnancy in certain areas of the body with exploring the resistance will release what ready, like anything, it is a journey back to self.

You always start from the ground up to create stability and connection to what you can feel and touch, the Earth. In your journey of yoga and movement connecting with a teacher that resonates with you. Understands this is powerful and creating a stable foundation that feels safe and nurturing means the nervous system will begin to trust in letting go. Light energy comes in through every Star Portal (chakra) of your bodysuit and from all corners of the Earth and in all directions of the winds. In any healing journey is it *key to feel safe and grounded first.*

For example, for those of you that have a fear of speaking and thinking that what you have to say doesn't matter. You may have been spoken over all of your life and often feeling others ignore what you have to say. If your throat or yoni is shut down and blocked, then the beauty is this is also where Your gift and power reside. There is a direct relationship between the 5th (Throat) and 2nd (Sacral) energy centre. As explored in *Wildflower,* the ability to orgasm and feeling free to moan in free expression and a healthy release is all connected. Healing of sexual shame, sexual trauma and the feminine power and innocence that has been fed off and manipulated to hook others. Over the years women's voices being shut down, unheard and spoken over and many times this is happening in your own family.

In contrast, the opposite is someone who 'over moans', which is very put on and fake, like porn is all a performance. The *performer bedroom program* reveals a deep-seated fear of letting go, being seen and feeling enough. Both are leaking valuable energy from the Chakra Star Portals/ Constellations.

This is not about wronging men as his feminine source power of creativity and imagination has been manipulated, raped and fed off my those seeking power, control and dominance and this began in childhood. To connect to the feminine source and the ability to dream and reclaim his disciplined action towards his chosen goals. To not settle by dropping into obedience and to stand along and protect the intuitive feminine and childlike innocence.

During sensual massage the freedom to moan effects the release of an orgasm and can assist many women who find reaching orgasm difficult. This also assists men to draw more energy into a heart that may feel wounded and to feel loved and acknowledged as a beautiful soul. There are many men that honesty is not being heard and given the respect and adoration that they deserve.

A chakra assists to determine how you experience life through your emotional reactions, desires and level of confidence. Let's explore these on a deeper level, starting from the ground up, it is time for *Root to Rise.*

As you explore this focus on the posterior of the body as the chakras are towards the back of the body. Feel the resonance of each chakra drawing you forward in life, like you have a gentle warm hand of encouragement that you can lean into and drawing your essence foreword. This is a Game changer!

Let's explore the 7-main chakras/Star portal constellations in the body. These are part of the 13 Star Constellations, Earth Star, in the Earth and above your crown, the Causal, Soul Star, Stellar Gateway and the Christ self.

MULADHARA

This is the 1st Chakra and is found at the Root/base of the spine. This is what assists you to be grounded and connected to the Earth. There is a connection between the nose and this chakra as it belongs to the Earth element, and this is directly related to smell. This has an impact on your nervous system and is associate with human survival. The Sanskrit word moola means 'root' or foundation, and this is exactly what this chakra is. Mooladhara is at the root of our chakra system and its influences are at the root of your entire existence.

Get grounded and rooted into the Earth to access inner strength. This is where your Kundalini Shakti that controls your instinct for food, survival, sleep and sex. The kundalini serpent sleeps coiled up until awakened to rise up 33-rung Jacob's ladder, of the spine. This is the Chakra of Tribe and the feeling of a sense of belonging. The path is not to hide in the tribe as even this security is an illusion which was created to produce the Socialised hive' mind of conditioning. It is your mission, if you accept it to be courageous to walk your own path into the wilderness away from the tribe. The explorer with curious childlike wonder. One of the easiest ways to begin to activate the 'Root Chakra' is by focusing the softened gaze at the tip of the nose.

Nose Tip Gazing

- Sit in an upright position with the spine lengthened, head upright, jaw relaxed
- Softly close the eyes and relax the whole body for 2-3 minutes
- Slowly crack open the eyes and softly gaze to the tip of the nose

- Do not strain, be gentle and breathing is relaxed.
- As the gaze softens, a double outline of the nose will appear
- These tow line converge at the tip of the nose, forming an inverted 'V'
- Concentrate on the apex of the 'V'
- The eyes may feel strained, the muscles strengthen, and it becomes softer
- Maintain a slow and steady gaze for a minute or more.
- Become aware of the breath, moving in and out through the nose
- Become aware at the same time of the sound of the breath
- Moving in and out of the nasal passages

- Become one with the practice,
- Awareness to the tip of the nose, the breath and the sound of the breath.
- Work up to 5 minutes never straining the eyes.
- End the practice by rubbing the palms together and then resting upon the closed eye sockets
- To relax and energise the eyes.

MULADHARA ACTIVATION

In a sitting position bring one of the heels of your foot and place it at your perineum. Place the heel in between the labia majora (outer) so there is an upward pressure to begin the awakening from the base up. There may be a slight pulsation and awakening, a stirring of sorts. Once you feel this bring the awareness up to the top of the vagina, to the back wall of the vagina near the cervix. This will become clearer once you are guided through the practice of Moola Bandha in Chapter 9.

Draw in and up and contract the inside of the vagina from the perineum upwards.

This is a key to raising consciousness - Z

- Element- Earth
- Star – Aquarius
- Colour - Red
- Sound- Lam

- Affirmation:

I am safe and connected, I am alive, and I am Earth.

- Postures: Utktasana- with pelvic tilt, Child's pose, Mountain pose, Tree pose, Seated postures and having one heal pressed into the perinium. Malasana with pelvic pulses and Cat /Cow posture (spine flexion/extension).

Mountain pose with lateral stretch

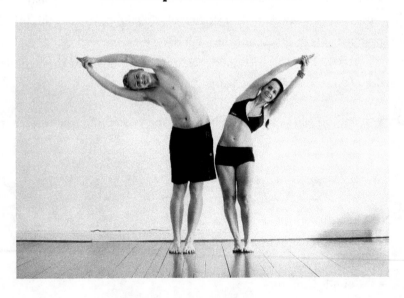

The Mountain pose is a great grounding postures to connect with the Earth and into a place of inner calm and peace. For fun see yourself standing like reeds in the river as you sway your upper body playfully side to side as if the water is moving you. As a kid you learnt to stand up and this was the beginning of being a conduit for Consciousness as the divine creative expression of you. You are Earthlings of the Earth and Light Houses for humanity.

Seated Twist with arm reach

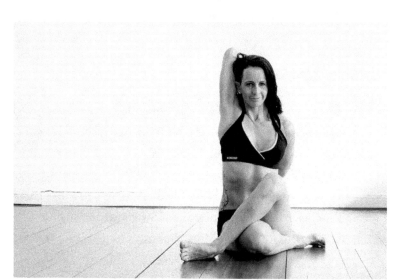

SVADHISTHANA

Svadhisthana is the 2nd Chakra located in the sacrum/ the centre of the pelvis and is known by some as the sacred water centre. It is the home of reproductive organs, sexual desires and creativity. A place where creativity and sensuality bubble up once awakened and stirred from the deep sleep.

This area is often taken over by the emotions and fear reactions.

The contraction and activation points are concerned with the genito-ovarian system in women.

Sahajoli, is the gentle contraction, and the contraction points being the clitoris, vaginal walls and urethra. This is a powerful practice to re-channel sexual energy and assist to awaken the second chakra, 'Swadhistana'. The nature of your second Chakra, Star/ energy wheel moves in *a fluid and spiral motion as water.* Knowing this, move your hips and pelvis in this way to assist the flow of healing lifeforce.

2ND CHAKRA LOCATION

- Sit in a comfortable position. Place one finger on the coccyx (the lowest part of the tailbone) and move up one inch or 2-3 cm
- Press into this area hard for 1 minute.
- When you remove the pressure, you will feel a residual sensation
- Bring your awareness to this residual sensation and move about one cm deep. This is the location of Swadhisthana chakra.
- Concentrate on it for two-three minutes and repeat the words mentally, Swadhisthana, Swadhisthana, Swadhisthana.

Opposing point of the 2nd Chakra to assist awakening

- Bring your awareness to the lower part of the abdomen and to the bony aspect at the front of the pelvis. This is known as the pubis and holds much sensual tension often from trauma.
- Press hard on this area for about one minute.

- The remove your fingers and concentrate on the point where your fingers were pressing.
- Repeat mentally, swadhisthana, swadhisthana, swadhisthana.

Now do the first 1st activation by *pressing both simultaneously* for about 1 minute really hard and as you release, *visualise a golden thread* and a magnetic pull between the two points. This is the *activation* of the 2nd Chakra taught in Kundalini Tantra.

You may notice a purification process with all these practices and sensitisation so ensure you are getting out in nature and grounding whilst incorporating physical movements into your day. This 2nd energy centre is where codependency, lust and sexual addictions play out. To shift is learning to have self-love practices, discipline rather than instant gratification and exploring the inner work without always replying on your partner. Meditation stimulates this area and awakens your healing ability, creativity, and sensual magnetism. It is all inter-related and can assist with the healing of sexual trauma and expressing your Truth.

This area of the body loves to move in a fluidity in cyclical patterns, circles, figure of eights and infinities.

- Element- Water
- Star – Capricorn
- Colour- Orange
- Sound- Vam

- Affirmation - I am flowing with ease, I am creative, I am dynamic, and I am sensual.

- Postures- Forward fold, Squat, Horse stance, and a Wide-leg fold. Pigeon, Warrior I, Warrior II and the Splits

Forward Fold

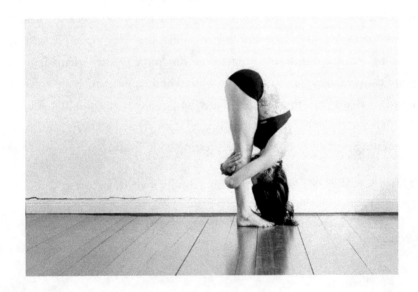

Modified wide- leg Straddle

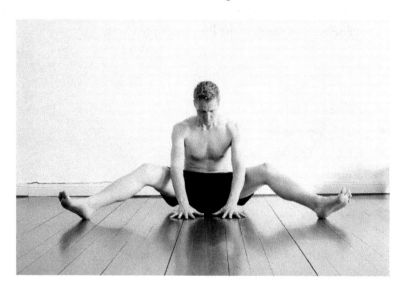

MANIPURA

Manipura is the 3rd Chakra and is found above the navel, at the solar plexus. It is associated with your digestive system and also your sense of the Self, the identity and ego (false self). This area is vital to awaken so that you can step into your truth and awaken your passion and purpose. It is associated with confidence and your *inner knowing and instinct,* the second brain of your *'gut instinct'*. It can reveal distortions in seeking power, control and dominance. To shift beyond this is to a path to shift beyond the labels and titles. It is a path to meeting your ego and pride and the path of humility beyond arrogance. An energy powerhouse that controls a huge amount of physical vitality. Think of the fire and passion in your belly and the butterflies you feel when you get nervous or intuition giving you a message to clarify through communicating what is being sensed. The excitement you feel, the more you awaken then the greater you feel.

It is a powerful source of energy and is often referred to as the Hara centre. A Star portal/doorway into all-knowing of all the wisdom of the body and a portal to generate and regulate the life force in the body.

- Element- Fire
- Star – Sagittarius
- Colour- Yellow
- Sound- Ram

- Affirmation- I am powerful, I am confident, I am worthy, and I am enough. I am humble.

- Postures- Boat, Seated twists, Core activation exercises.

Assisted Boat

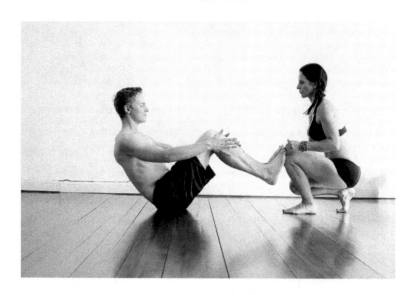

Full Boat Pose

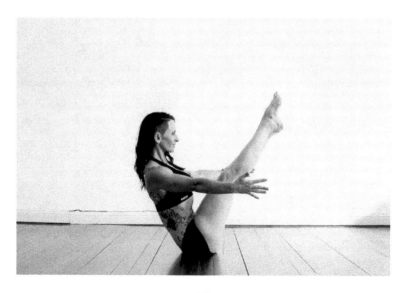

There is a Solar Star constellation between the 3rd and 4th energy chakra wheels. This is the Star constellation of Scorpio and is golden in nature.

ANAHATA

Anahata is the 4th Chakra and is found at the centre of the chest and heart. This is the most powerful of the chakras and is associated with the lungs and the elements of air. For many this is blocked or closed off to protect the heart, as it is a place of vulnerability and the sacred hearts truth. I see client's postures hunched over at the beginning of working together and from the flat words that they choose.

It takes a willingness to be brave and courageous to allowing an opening with trust. It requires, letting go of the past, and forgiveness moment to moment. Once this is opened, life takes on a new level of meaning. This is the area of love, compassion and forgiveness. Once opened the heart is infinite and over-flowing, and the doorway to realms beyond and it is the portal to begin to walk the path of heaven on Earth.

It is through the upper heart of the Thymus that the student as the explorer of self can access realms beyond and into higher states of consciousness of playing the infinite game.

- Element- Air
- Star – Libra & Alpha Centauri
- Colour- Green and Magenta Pink
- Sound- Yam

- Affirmations- I am kind, I am love and I am opening even more. I trust, I forgive, and I am loved.

- Postures- Camel, Bridge, Wheel, Backbends and Triangle

Camel

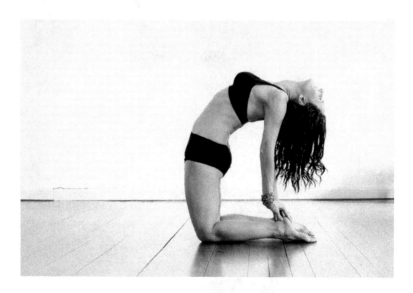

Unsupported Camel

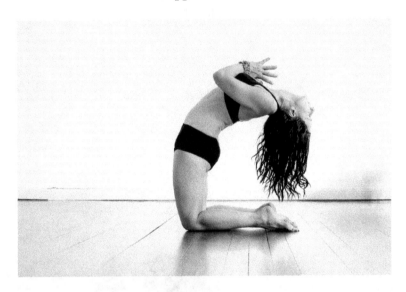

Bridge

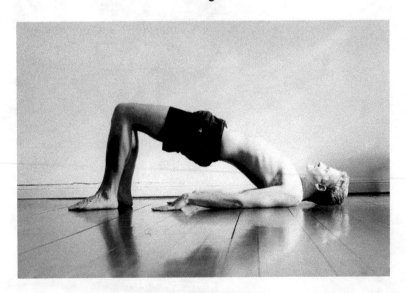

Assisted Bow

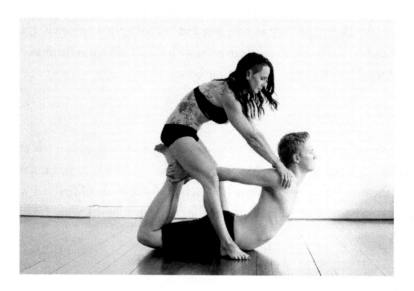

The assisted bow is a beautiful stretch to do with a partner. This is about communicating through words, breath and touch, being present and learning how to work together. Allow the one being stretched to come into the bow position and then holding your own body weight, lower your bottom softly and slowly onto their feet. Make sure their toes are flexed otherwise you will end up with toes up your bottom! My upper body posture is not so great in this picture so be aware when supporting postures to assist not hold and place your own sacred bodysuit at risk of injury.

Slowly reach the outside of their shoulders and gently sit more weight onto their feet. Get them to breathe into their heart space and upper chest. The assist more with tight hips that will restrict the movement of back bending, place a bolster or rolled mat or cushion under the hips, in line with the pubic bone. Enjoy the journey of partner work. This also opens the throat centre, which is connected to your free and unapologetic expression. It also presses onto the pubic bone so can assist with the 2nd chakra as many bodies hold trauma and tension in the pubic bone!

By yourself, grab a large pillow or bolster and lay back onto it, so it is resting down the length of your spine. Open up your arms wide as you can and breathe into the places that feel stuck, chest, front of shoulders and with the breath soften and relax. Stay here for five-ten minutes with the neck supported.

MORE HEART OPENING

Stand facing a wall, reach arms up above the ears, shoulder height, press palms into the wall, bend the knees and soften the chest down towards to floor. This will create an opening through the front of the shoulders, chest and open this center. Stay here and breathe and when you start to lose the breath, trust you are pushing too hard and all you have to do is ease off! Here is a floor variation, where the floor is what would be the wall.

Tip: draw the pubic bone towards the hips so that the lower back arch flattens to protect the lower back. The focus is on opening the shoulders and thoracic and not the lower back!

Anahatasana

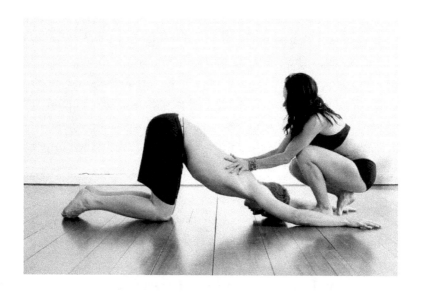

Reverse Plank

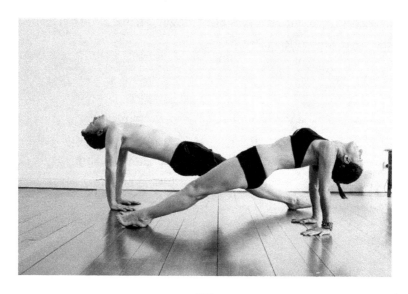

VISUDDHA

Visuddha is the 5th Chakra: This is found in the throat and centre of the neck and is called the energetic home of expressing through speaking, sound and superpowers of clairaudient hearing capabilities and the throat houses your endocrine glands. Think of this as the area of communication. This helps you to express and expand your conversation to the divine higher power. To open up the throat centre will assist in the purification of the entire system.

For many, this has been shut down and suppressed and as mentioned there is a strong correlation with sensual pleasure and the freedom to express during intimacy. This may have been shut down from an early age, from feeling not heard and being hushed by our well-meaning parents' or teachers'. This gets shut down in the wounded inner masculine in women where they then become bossy and over controlling of others. This is why not expressing your intuitive sensing of the gut can make you feel nauseous, express what you are feeling.

You actually have another G-spot deep in the throat that is stimulated when giving oral pleasure to a man and when stimulated can lead to an orgasm in the one performing oral sex. There are magical things that can happen by opening the throat, and again, this requires trust, openness and raw vulnerability to be curious.

- Element- Ether
- Star – Virgo
- Colour- Turquoise/Sky blue
- Sound- Ham

- Affirmations- I am empowered, what I have to say is important, I speak with conviction, and I am honest.

- Postures- Fish, Camel, Shoulder stand and Lions Breath

Shoulder Stand

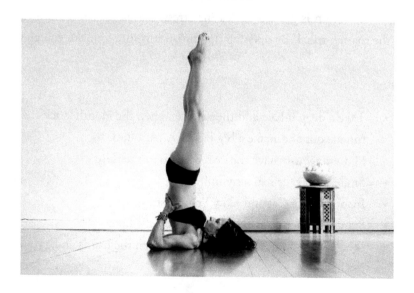

Lions' Breath

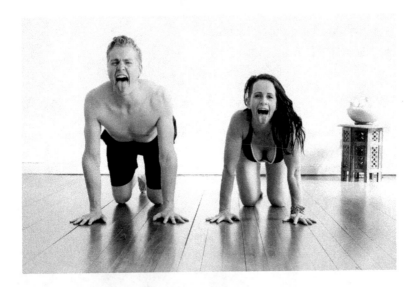

The Lions Breath is great for releasing stress, sensual tension, and brings out the roaring tribal. By opening the throat, it is sure to make you giggle!

- Take a deep inhale and then exhale, open the mouth, stick the tongue out and make a big HAAAAAA sound.
- Simultaneously have the eyes gaze up to the third eye.
- Smile as this feels super yum!
- Incorporate a Cat and Cow Yoga posture.
- Start on all fours, knees and hands on the floor
- Inhale, round out the back, press through the hands and gaze at the belly.

- Then, exhale sink the chest to the floor, tip the seat bones away and as you exhale into lion's breath.
- Repeat, a minimum of three.

AJNA

Ajna is the 6th Chakra, the third eye, above and behind the eyebrows. This is the command centre within the mid brain. This is the meeting point between Ida (feminine) and Pingala (Masculine) Nadis, lines of energy channels within the body. It is where the mind and body join one another. This is associated with the Pituitary Gland. It is the pituitary gland that secretes two important hormones- oxytocin and vasopressin. Oxytocin is nurturing, sexual pleasure and love hormone. Vasopressin regulates circadian rhythms- sleep cycles and reabsorption back into the blood stream.

The pituitary is important for pineal gland activation. Alternate nostril breathing will help to balance this centre and assist in your meditation practice. Insight, intuition, dreaming, visions and inner wisdom. The alternate nostril breathing will also assist with the 2nd Chakra energy, you can lightly tap the area in between the eyebrows to wake it up.

- Element- Light
- Star – Leo, Orion & Sirius
- Colour- Indigo/midnight blue
- Sound- Kasham

- Affirmations- I am connecting and trusting in my inner wisdom, I am seeing, observing as the I am witness.
- Postures – Headstand, Rabbit, Child's pose, meditation.

Child's Pose

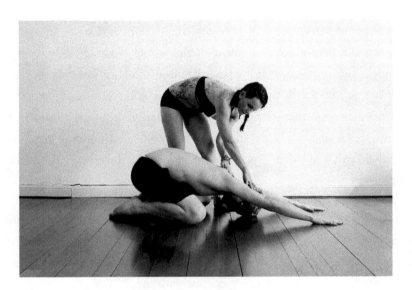

Posture

Rest your forehead and roll out the back of the neck and gently massage place between the eyebrows that is pressing into the floor; this is the area of the third eye, Ajna centre. Here, in the picture I am getting a client to relax his shoulders with the touch of my hands. His knees are wide, so that his head can come down to the floor. For those that are tight in the hips and the head is a long way from the floor, place a block, cushion or some books under the forehead. This will bring the floor to meet the forehead and to maintain alignment always modify when required. This is the perfect position to restore the nervous system into relaxation and inner balance.

SRI YANTRA – 3RD EYE OPENING

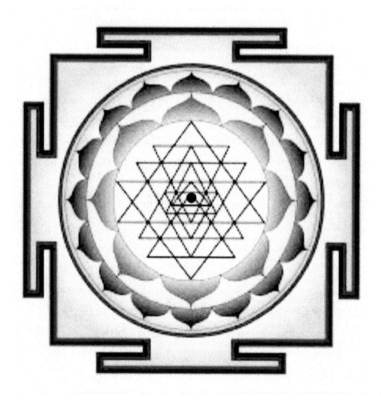

A complex sacred geometry consisting of 9- interlocking triangles and used in the Shri Vidya School of Hinduism. It is used for as an instrument, meaning Yantra in Sanskrit. You can focus upon the red dot (black dot in this case), which symbolises the central point, referred to as Bindu.

The triangles represent the cosmos and the human body.

Focus upon the triangle around the black dot, the 4th one facing down so the chalice or cup opening is facing upwards with the apex of the triangle pointing down. Gaze at the symbol with a gentle yet soft gaze, slowly begin to close your eyes and the symbol will begin to arise over time in your mind's eye. This I will often focus upon during my meditation practice.

This will assist to purify, open and clear inner seeing

SHAMBHAVI MUDRA – EYEBROW GAZING

- Sit in a meditation posture that you feel comfortable in.
- Spine is lengthened, hands resting upon the thighs, palms facing down
- Look forwards at a fixed point, then look upwards as high as possible without moving your head.
- Focus the eyes and concentrate on the eyebrow centre.
- Try to allow thoughts to be held suspended in bubbles
- Meditate upon ajna - the space between your eyebrows.
- Repeats the sound 'OM... as AUM' with awareness and feel the resonance and vibration within the ajna centre. Keep the mantra short, a few seconds followed by the next OM.
- Repeat for 3-5 mins
- Then be still and hear the Universal sound in the Ajna Center.

TRATAKA MEDITATION - INNER SEEING

Out of the main five senses, sight is arguably the most powerful. In order to perceive through touch or taste, we need to be in contact with the object. In order to perceive a smell or sound, we need to be near the source of that smell or sound. However, with our eyes we can perceive objects and landscapes miles away, without actually being there. Indeed, 80% of all sensory data we process comes through our vision (source). After the brain, your eyes are the most complex organ in the body, containing more than 200 million working parts. They are also the fastest muscle in your body, and can function at 100% at any given moment, without needing to rest.

What is the meaning of Trataka?

Trataka is a meditation technique which involves focusing the eyes (and, in turn, the mind) through intent but relaxed gazing. There are many ways of doing Trataka and candle gazing is just one of them. In all forms of trataka you can integrate breath awareness or the repetition of a mantra if you find it helpful, although it's not commonly taught this way.

BENEFITS:

- Improves concentration, memory, and willpower
- Improves visualisation skills
- Improves cognitive function
- Cures eye diseases
- Makes the eyes stronger, clearer, and brighter
- Helps with insomnia
- Clears accumulated mental/emotional complexes
- Brings suppressed thoughts to the surface

- Increases nervous stability
- Calms the anxious mind

AWARENESS

- Honour your body and do not force
- Listen to the messages of the body
- Apply 'Tiger balm' to the 3rd eye to assist
- Massage the '3rd eye' to stimulate
- Clear choices in life = Clearer Seeing

SAHASARA

Sahasara is the 7th Chakra and is found at the crown at top of the head. This is also associated with the pineal gland. Its position is at the centre of the brain, behind and above the pituitary gland. The pineal gland is cone shaped, like the Fibonacci sequence. This shape symbolises growth and unifying force for all creation. This is our connection to our higher self, consciousness and God and Living your truth. As you evolve the energy will start to move up the spine and into this centre.

- Element- Thought
- Star – Cancer
- Colour- Violet or white
- Sound- Om
- Affirmations- I am God, I am the Goddess, I am that I am.
- Postures- Headstand, downward facing dog and ½ Lotus

This next posture is fun to explore with an adjustment. Only do this when you feel comfortable with placing weight through your shoulders and onto your hands. Firstly, come into DWFD (downward facing dog) and very gently bring one foot up a time onto others the sacrum, either side of the spine and never on the spine. Feet turned out onto each side of the spine. The one in DWFD bends their knees to lift and tilt their sit bones up to the sky.

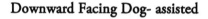

This builds trust, communication and a deeper offering.

Downward Facing Dog- assisted

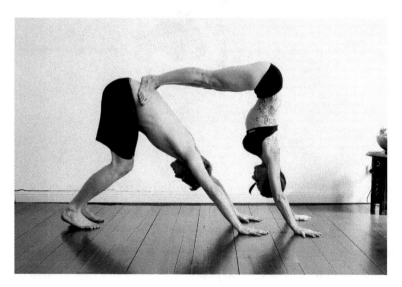

Headstand

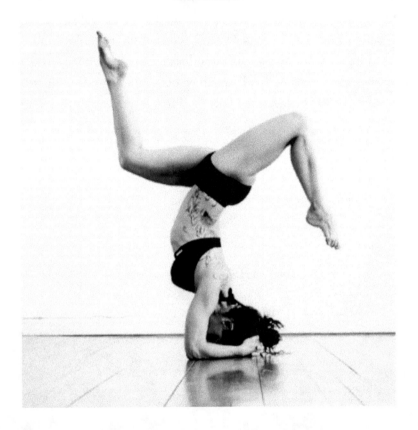

The Headstand *Sirsasana* is a great way to activate your crown chakra as it helps to put pressure onto the top of your head. This encompasses everything that is beyond your linear as well as personal needs. Even if you cannot do a headstand (yet!), you can sit on a chair, with your legs wide and allow your torso to rest down between your legs and your head to hang loose towards the floor. Place a pillow of a pile of books on the floor to rest the crown of the head down as this will stimulate your crown. This is a secret to longevity, beauty and brings an immediate sense of calm and inner peace. It clears the mind and balances the soul. To close your eyes is to go deeper within and trust in being supported by the Universe. Stay here for as long as you can, work up to 5-minutes for a daily beauty tip and a secret to staying young!

The Chakra has a seed sound that resonates with its centre and powerful to integrate in with each posture, explore and play!

These specific sounds balance that centre and this is a powerful exercise that anyone can do. Yoga is an inward journey back to the self, the learning never ends, life and relationships with self and others is yoga! These were the seed sounds covered with each of the chakras, go back over them and explore whilst in the postures.

Om is the universal sound within the universe, sounded as AUM. You see the word at the beginning of these three-words that encompass all that is, the divine God consciousness.

- Omnipotent- unlimited power and able to do anything
- Omniscience- a state of knowing everything
- Omnipresence- The presence of God/ The Divine everywhere

The calling out of the sounding of Om, at the beginning and the end of a practice is the doorway into the unknown.

AUM- Meditation is the constant contemplation of That- OSHO

CHAPTER 9: ORGASM AND THE COSMIC ORGASM

"Expose yourself to your deepest fear, after that, fear has no power, and the fear of freedom shrinks and vanishes." -Jim Morrison

ORGASM AND THE MENTAL MIND

The key to a woman's sexual desire and pleasure centres is through mental stimulation from her partner. To say what you desire and adore and for the man to tell her what he desires about her, and how you are going to ravish her. This goes deep into her sub-conscious part of the mind and the courage to explore the emotional depths of being human. The more open you are, the more freely the communication flows as too will her orgasms. She needs to feel safe in herself to fully open in full trust and to hear a man she loves willing to be vulnerable and share from his raw heart.

The cosmic orgasm is where You are heading, and is a moment-to-moment psychic awareness to a now state of presence Zoe Bell

Many are chasing orgasms to experience an empty release and a draining of life-force energy. Connection, intimacy and harnessing the energy are key for whole-body orgasm and most of society are stuck in their genitals and addictions of ignorance.

'A powerful force of intense orgasm comes from a sweeping, sensuous takeover of the mind followed by a guiltless release of psychosexual emotions. The mind takeover is a sensationally unique experience that serves the profoundly beneficial and needed psychological function of letting the individual know that this concrete and real experience is the reward for living a rational and productive life. Intense orgasm is also the symbol that a person is living the way he or she, as a biological organism, is deigned to live. In joy'
Zoe Bell

An explosive orgasm for both the man and woman is a visibly powerful experience. An intense orgasm is more of psychological experience than a physical one, that can range from calm to violently explosive. While many have experienced physically explosive orgasm, far fewer of experienced psychologically intense orgasms. This orgasm absorbs both the mind and the body. It is a magical experience to ride the orgasmic wave together, and lose yourselves within one another, where two souls are so present with one another that they shift dimensions. Thus, creating a portal of bliss of souls intertwining in an experience of ecstatic bliss.

Sexuality beyond the pure physical act is the dance with the divine cosmos and a path to higher states of consciousness.

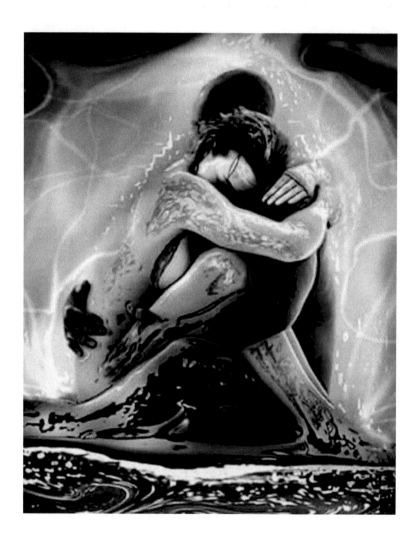

Here are is the difference between the tension buildup and the tension release. Referenced from The Potent Threesome- Mark Hamilton.

VARIABLES CONTROLLING ORGASMISTIC FORCE

The difference Between Tension Buildup and Tension Release

Creation of Sexual Tension   Release of Sexual Tension

Creation of Sexual Tension	Release of Sexual Tension
• Physical Stimulation	• Relaxation
• Psychological Stimulation	• Freedom
• Imagination	• Guiltlessness
• Fantasies	• Fearlessness
• Control	• Joyfulness
• Discipline	• Openness
• Sexual Partner	• Sexual partner
• Self-esteem	• Self-esteem
• Self-confidence	• Self-confidence

The explosiveness of the orgasm is not only a function of the tension, differential before and after orgasm release, but it is function of how fast the tension is released. The importance of the sexual partner having healthy self-esteem and self-confidence is vital in creating sexual tension, and also the release phase. To fully release is to feel free, guiltless pleasure and openness, and the esteem for self, so choose wisely.

The orgasm is not the end goal either as we will explore deeper. Using the orgasm to release tension is not the healthiest way to let go as it will only release temporary tension and not the entire pleasure bodysuit.

Attraction to your partner is vital.

Yes, the mental mind connection is vital so too is the physical attraction and primal smell to the other. It is a nervous system that will also attract a Soul as you awaken you will become more selective as each soul you are intimate with as mentioned previously in Wildflower you will take on their Karma. It is about being attracted to them as a spiritual being and respecting them as a Soul, proud of them and holding in the highest of loving regard, attraction has so many layers. The magnetic pull has to be experienced, as words cannot describe it with the beauty that it deserves the body needs to purr by being within one another's presence.

THE MIND DURING ORGASM

Normal State

The mind is clear. No interference patterns. Both long-term and short-term thinking processes are functioning and there are no states of pleasure.

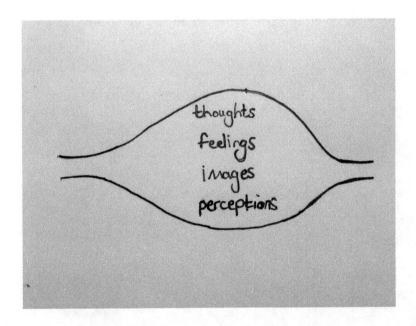

Ordinary Orgasm

There are a few sexual patterns interfering with or partially blocking normal contents of the mind. The ability to think shrinks to be more in the here and now moment of sexual pleasure.

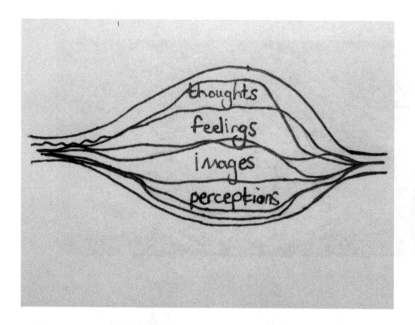

Intense Orgasm

To visualise intense orgasm, there is no thought, perceptions disappear, all that exists is squeezed out of existence of the conscious mind. No thought, where the thinking process ceases. Totality of mind only focuses on the pleasure of intense orgasm.

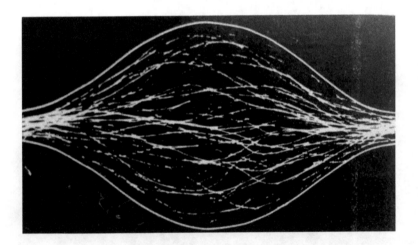

Most souls are stuck in the orgasm, blowing their load to feel relief, knocking out orgasms to feel a connection, and yet, left feeling drained and empty. Mindlessly fucking to soothe the numbness within and no conscious awareness of mind, body and Spirit. It takes individual discipline, conscious thought and immense control to take this into the sacredness of Union between two souls, where orgasm is not the destination. A path to deepen the love connection through the heart and experience joy, bliss and eternity of interconnecting into a union with the divine cosmos of higher states of ecstasy. The Egyptians were master's when it came to sensuality and orgasming for longevity. Isis and Osiris were masters in this sensual magiKal dance of pure devotion.

THE IMPORTANCE OF ORGASM

Taken from an article by Drunvalo Melchizedek, December 15, 2015, printed in Conscious Sexuality Secrets.

"The ancient Egyptians believed that orgasm is more than just something that feels good and allows procreation. They believed an orgasm is sacred and that is the energy of an orgasm is harnessed in the right way, it would become a source of infinite pranic energy and thus lead to eternal life."

The Egyptians were wise masters of sensuality and they believed then an orgasm is sacred. Here are some of the beneficial effects of the orgasm.

- *Helps to Prevent Physical and Emotional Disease*

According to the Egyptians the release during orgasm will release dysfunctional energy form the body which can thus assist in preventing disease from manifesting.

- *Helps Raise Consciousness*

They believed that an orgasm was the doorway to access the higher chakras and under the right conditions will allow a person to begin the process towards enlightenment. This process will lead to higher levels of consciousness and into the world beyond his plane.

- *Increases Strength & Vitality*

They believed that an orgasm can make your stronger, more alive, revitalising relationships as more life force energy is flowing through you, and this may lead you to eternal life.

Drunvalo, goes on to explain that many people become ignorant to what happens to their bodies after orgasm. According to the ancient Traditions such as the Hindu, Tibetan, Tantric and the Taoist the orgasmic energy moves up the spine and out the top of the head.

In a few rare cases the energy is released down the spine below the feet. In both cases – the concentrated life-force-prana energy is dissipated and lost to the ground, like discharging a battery.

He goes on to add, that the world's Tantric system that he is aware of believe that orgasm with ejaculation brings one a little bit closer to death, as they lose their vital life force, so many of these systems avoid ejaculation of even avoid sexual inter course believing it increases their consciousness. The Egyptians found that not to be the case

"Egyptians believe orgasms are healthy and necessary including the release of sperm in males, and that the sexual energy must be controlled in a deeply esoteric procedure that is unlike any other system"

They believed that when this energy is controlled, the human orgasm becomes a source of infinite pranic energy that is not lost. They believed that the entire light body, known as *Mer-Ka-Ba* surrounding the body benefits from this sexual release. The *Ankh* is a key. This we will explore after looking at the Merkaba. The Pleiades were also master's in sacred sensuality as mentioned in Wildflower.

MER-KA-BA

Merkaba, pronounced Mer-Ke-Bah, is the divine light vehicle allegedly used by ascended masters to connect with and reach those in tune with the higher realms. *'Mer'* means special kind of light. *'Ka'* means spirit. *'Ba'* means body and interpretations of reality according to the Egyptians. Mer-Ka-Ba means the spirit and body surrounded by counter-rotating fields of light, (wheels within wheels), spirals of energy as in DNA, which transports spirit and body from one dimension to another.

In Hebrew it means vehicle and is spelt Merkabah.

We have millions and trillions of MerKaBa, it is what makes up all space. Your body are toroidal energetic fields of constantly flowing energy. It is what you are and that is why when getting into nature you feel more alive and vibrant as there are less distractions to feel into this powerful force field of energy.

In 2017, I was drawn to teachers of light language, facilitators of energy, and sought guidance from Psychic's, Healers and Shamans. Learning, integrating the teachings daily with intuition the DNA began to awaken and upgrade from within. Each teacher you are drawn to and work with are keys to awaken a piece of the puzzle to awaken your unique Soul codes. When you have the pieces and diligently apply and integrate the practices you get to create your own unique puzzle and gifts to access as the creative expression and embodied emergence.

When you are asking for guidance, be ready to receive as the teacher(s) will find you!

Let's explore the Mer-Ka-Ba and dive deeper into the sacred connection within intimacy and sensual union between two souls. When two souls are connecting their light bodies in an intimate setting and are able to become aware of their MerKaBa activation, breath regulation with activation of the energy channels of the Ida, Pingala and Sushumna, magic happens. It is then those intimate states of higher frequency are accessed and reached. The focus is no longer on orgasm, it is about dancing within the Universal forces and Cosmic orgasmic states that building upon the life-force field for the greater good for humanity.

Love is your natural state of consciousness, there is no past, there is no future, it is all happening within the now.

When two souls collide and dissolve into one a state of bliss and eternity is experienced, where time pauses. A morphing of time, as time is another illusion of the Maya. To truly experience this, you have to be experienced this with a soul who can guide you with crystal clear commands of love.

Past-Present-future

There is no meeting. Only lovers meet because suddenly when you are present with a soul, a different time comes into existence. Both meet in a single moment, and the moment neither belongs to you, or your lover. This is something new. Neither out of your past, or your lovers of past. Time in the moment moves present to present, a meeting of two present moments and higher dimensions reveal. The dimension of eternity never ends. It has no future, and it has no past.

"It is present
Here, and now
Potency of presence
A drop in the ocean of existence"

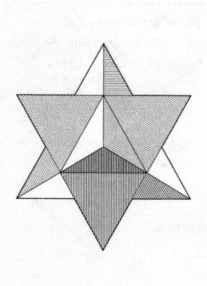

Researcher and physicist Drunvalo Melchizedek describes this figure as a 'Star Tetrahedron' since it can be viewed as a three-dimensional Star of David. By imagining two superimposed 'Star Tetrahedrons' as counter rotating, along with specific 'Prana' breathing techniques, certain eye movements and mudras, it is taught that one can activate a non-visible 'saucer' shaped energy field around the human body that is anchored at the base of the spine. Depending on the height of the person doing the exercise, this field is about 55 feet across once activated, this 'saucer' shaped field is capable of carrying one's consciousness directly to higher dimensions.

The MerKaBa is an inter-dimensional vehicle consisting of two equally sized, interlocked tetrahedra of light with a common centre, where one tetrahedron points up and the other down. This point symmetric form is called a Stella octangular or stellated octahedron which can also be obtained by extending the faces of a regular octahedron until they intersect again. The upper tetrahedra represents the masculine energy and the bottom upside down tetrahedral represents the feminine. The masculine spins clockwise and the feminine anti-clockwise.

There are many ways to activate the MerKaBa, and this is the way that I have learnt and integrate into this vessel. This can be done sitting or standing, it is all personal preference, begin with sitting. Here is the difference between the Mer-Ka-Ba in woman and man. The instructions below still follow as guided.

WOMAN   *MAN*

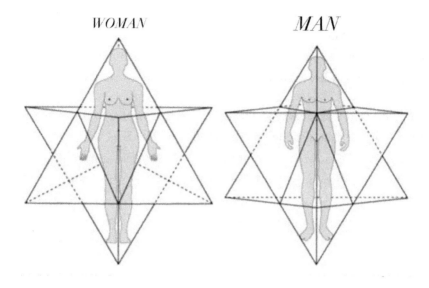

Firstly, you have to clear out the central channel - Sushumna, so bring your awareness to connect with the Earth Star, deep in the core of Mother Earth, and imagine this silver energy coming up from mother earth into your root (chakra 1) chakra, and penetrating the 1st, 2nd, 3rd energy centres until it reaches the heart (4th centre). Next, connect with the Soul star, which is about 6-8 inches above your crown. Imagine golden light streaming down and into the crown, through the head, throat and into the heart space. Imagine these energies clearing out the central Channel of any debris, to bring the connection into the heart space. Stay here, until it feels crystal clear.

Next, bring awareness to the male energy from the star Sirius streaming down and filling the chalice of the Soul Star, filling up with its energy, and streaming through the crown and into the heart space, this energy then begins to activate the upper tetrahedron, as the masculine tetrahedron begins to spin in a clockwise position, from left to right. Imagine it begin to spin really fast left to right.

Next, bring the awareness to the star constellation of Orion, the female energy of the stars, filling up the chalice of the Soul Star, and then penetrating the crown, throat and into the heart. Activating the bottom tetrahedron to begin to spin in an anti-anti-clockwise direction, right to left. Imagine it staining really fast, whilst the masculine space is spinning in a clockwise direction really fast.

Your body may rock, move and this is a powerful activation. Make sure to ground with your feet upon the earth. Each Chakra/Star portal is a MerKaBa and each of these points an infinity.

Here is a picture of a couple bringing this into sacred union, this is something you are guided through and an aspect to what I teach to couples in Sacred Sensuality. This is magical to bring into a sacred union between souls. This can be explored without any penetration and with a friend, to understand the energy and practice and connecting in a sensual and loving union of the life force energies.

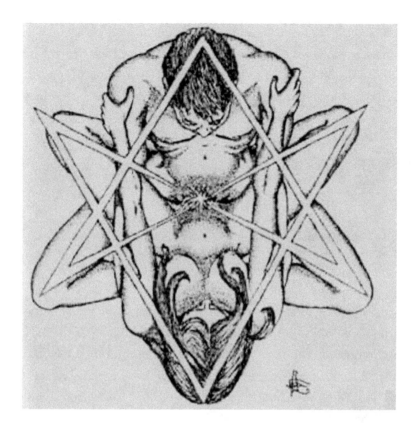

THE ANKH

The Ankh is known as the key of life, *Crux Ansata,* Egyptian cross. It represents the union of male and female Gods, Osiris and Isis, and the alliance of Earth to Sky. The cross aspect being the symbol of life, and the circle, a symbol of eternity. The staff of the cross is like the spine, representing the energetic channel of Sushumna, where the masculine and feminine forces of energy intertwine and flow. A powerful symbol as a pathway deeper into sacred union with intimacy with that special other and also the sacred union within self.

The key to the Divine to access higher wisdom and a doorway to unleash superpowers from within. There are many meanings, and many cultures and religions will have the Ankh within their symbols. Symbols are powerful, when linked with the potency of breath union, soul to soul intimate connection through the eyes, *'windows of the soul'* and awareness of the electromagnetic forces within the channels of Ida, Pingala and Sushumna.

This is a *sacred sensual union of bliss.*

The Ankh represents the pathway of the flow of sensual life force energy in sacred union, so that the energy keeps building and is not lost through the crown in orgasm. This takes practice alone, before enjoying this with your partner. The area in the centre at the bottom of the loop is the heart centre. As the individual is reaching orgasm, this surge of sensual energy is pushed out of the body, projected out of the heart, a big breath is inhaled in through the nose, around 80% and held, and this energy is moved with awareness in a curved shape, upwards and through the crown centre and then down the back of the body and into the heart centre.

This final part of the hoop of the descent from crown to heart, the rest of the breath is drawn into the body, and as it reaches the heart exhaled slowly. While exhaling the sensual energy is drawn back down to the sacral chakra, and a holding of presence with one another. In stillness, communicating only through the eyes and deep soul to soul messages.

It is then that you open up your hearts and become bathed in one another's infinite love. This can be repeated many times reaching ecstatic levels of bliss, where orgasm is secondary and not the destination. This takes practice alone at first, until one can learn to play with the energy, as it does not happen over-night.

Making love face to face with your partner brings a deeper level of intimacy, as you are able to kiss and dive deep into one another's eyes creating alchemy because two hearts are interlocking their magnetic field increasing their life force energy. This is the power of magnetism between two people and is a fundamental component to the cosmic vibration of love.

Your bodies energy is transformed through the magnetic field of the heart and the all-knowing star portal of the navel.

YOUR NAME HAS A V-IBRATION

My Soul mission became clearer once I embraced my birth name, Zoe.

Rebecca and Becky for short is my second name and Anna my third name. Rebecca means to tie, to bind, to snare, a noose, and from reading *'Breaking Free',* it makes sense and another piece of the Soul suffocation to breaking free of shame and finding my voice.

I am grateful as it was the perfect name to unravel the mystery, heal lifetimes of karma, and learn vital lessons to share a path with direct inner-standing. It was on my 44th Birthday that I made it known to those in my circle that I was going to be using my birthname. Zoe, means life, abundant life, MerKaBa, 5th Dimension, Goddess and is another translation of the name Eve. Anna means Grace. It was around this time that the Ankh was brought into my awareness and life shifted.

From researching my name on She Knows dot com I found that the Soul Expression of Zoe is a 1, and the Soul Urge is an 11.

I was born on 1st November, (1.11) at 11:11 am. 11:11 is significant as it is known as *The Awakening Code.* A time of synchronicities to be present enough to notice.

Soul Urge: Number 11

People with this name have a deep inner desire to inspire others in a higher cause, and to share their own strongly held views on spiritual matters.

Soul Expression: Number: 1

People with this name tend to initiate events to be leaders rather than followers, with powerful personalities. They tend to be focused on specific goals, experience a wealth of creative new ideas, and have the ability to implement these ideas with efficiency and determination. They tend to be courageous and sometimes aggressive. As unique, creative individuals, they tend to resent authority, and are sometimes stubborn, proud, and impatient.

Bell has great significance as JFK had the Bell in many of his pictures and inscribed on the Bell of his yacht. The Bell represents a calling in of remembrance and the 11^{th of} November at 11 am is Remembrance Day, honoured with a 1-minute silence.

'Where one goes, we all go' – JFK

Soul messages are all around you, and you will see them when you are in a place of asking and ready to seek deeper meaning. It depends on what your RAS (Reticular Activation system) and emotional guidance system is putting out, as the Universe will deliver.

Perhaps, pause and explore the different meanings, messages, soul urge and soul expression within your name. If your name given at birth no longer aligns then seek guidance on changing it. Letters create numbers, everything is a sequence of numbers, and all numbers have a vibration of energy.

Your mission is to radiate and activate the remembrance of the light within. This is felt as *Peace, Love & Harmony.*

A POTENT JEWEL WITHIN

There is a place within that once you access it will restore your energy, stir and awaken the Kundalini life-force energy and raise your consciousness. It brings you to a very calm, connected and centred place. Within the body there are three bandhas which are dormant.

- *Jalandhara bandha - situated in the throat*
- *Uddiyana - situated in the abdomen*
- *Moola bandha - situated in the perineum.*

Moola means *'root'*, and *'Source of all creation'*, and bandha means *'lock'* within the body that the yogis incorporate into yoga practice. This lock prevents the downwards movement of energy, which naturally falls back down due to gravity, and is vital to keep this powerful life-giving energy within the container, the body. It is the activation of these three-bandhas that awakens Kundalini energy and enters the central channel, Sushumna (The Middle way)

To physically describe all three, moola bandha is the conscious, willful contraction of the perineum/cervix, Uddiyana bandha of the solar plexus and Jalandhara bandha of the throat. This physical awareness can then have the potential after disciplined and willful practice will shift into psychic activation through awareness, of moola bandha.

This contraction and squeezing of muscles of the perineal, abdominal and cervical (neck) muscles is the mechanics behind the bandhas.

The one explored for the purpose of Soul Codes is moola bandha. This has a direct impact on the nervous system and brings calm to the body, lowering blood pressure, with a sense of deep rest and relaxation. And the stimulation of the energy on the first chakra, Mooladhara, and an awakening of the kundalini energy. This energy is the life-force, life renewing energy, which is sensual in nature. This is also the jewel to activate when visualising your dreams and desires. It builds up and awakens the dormant sensual energy within. And will assist in the ability to be present within all relationships and strengthen your connection.

Moola Bandha

The activation is different for men and women. This is a basic explanation as requires instruction with a yoga teacher that has mastered this practice themselves over years. I say this with discernment as you dive in deeper with each new awareness being implemented with guidance of the body work and moola therapy. Like anything and everything, it is a journey, and each step is vital to integrate. This will begin the process as many will read through this and never book the time into integrate and practice it, why?

Most souls are habitual with a line of excuses. Nothing will change until you choose to be the change, and when you think you know, you miss the teaching before you, as arrogance is blocking clear seeing.

For men to activate this area, it begins with gently contracting the perineum, the area of skin between the asshole and the balls, like you are lifting your balls up. A magical jewel, that is a few cm's in. There is a drawing up and in, as the energy begins to stir. Begin with contracting for 3-5 seconds and the relax. Allow this time to build up to 10 seconds and then relax. The relaxation is vital in order to let go. This can be great to activate at the point near orgasm and holding, to cycle the energy as in the Ankh looping of sensual energy. The purpose here is to 'switch on, wake-up' as this energy is creative in nature.

For women, the area to contract is at the top end of the posterior wall of the vagina, near the cervix. The contraction is a drawing up and back. Initially this will feel like nothing, so persevere and seek the guidance of a teacher, with the yoni sensual massage, or exploring with one of your fingers deep inside. After practicing for a while this will shift into a psychic contraction and no physical contraction of the muscles. This is magical way to create a vaginal orgasm and milk his lingam inside the yoni. When holding at the point of orgasm, ease off and breath with your partner, eyes contact is vital to stay connected and heart to heart, it is often best for a woman to be on top. As I am writing my moola bandha is bubbling and pulsating, and I feel instant calm and bliss.

This is a very different exercise to Kegel pelvic floor exercises I would highly recommend this inner energy practice of drawing up rather than pressing down and the pressure leaking out of the vagina. This is an ideal practice for women that have had POP, Pelvic Floor Prolapse and to prevent POP. Pushing down and your vagina dropping to the floor is horrific and a story shared by a dear soul sister.

Practice the moola bandha contraction at home, hold for 3-5 seconds and the relax. Repeat this and build up to holding for 10 seconds. Practice throughout the day whenever you remember.

This activation will at first increase the urge to have sex, this is the kundalini energy as it natural wakes and stirs you up. The lower animalistic urges of lust will take over and then you begin to one day explore a deeper connection by building this energy up as you don't want to keep leaking this life-force giving energy. This shifting of the energy will bring it towards the heart and to the higher chakras, for insight, clarity and intuition.

Orgasms will deepen in intensity and love making becomes a spiritually powerful experience for both.

There is a mad rush of many seeking enlightenment, in a rush to get somewhere. You are born enlightened and then you forgot, and your life is about Soul remembrance. This is a process of being able to follow a sequence of practices, training alongside a teacher to be guided in a foundational way (meaning a soul who has mastered self and what they preach and live by is what they teach). I am the embodiment and emergence of all that I teach and now it is second nature.

It is not a race, the spiritual path is about taking it slow so on can integrate and purify, mind, body and spirit. The nervous system needs time to adapt to adjust to the new energy, kundalini-life giving force within. Nourish each practice with loving care and the path will be much smoother, as when you push and force, then universe will push back as a process of rebalancing. These practices all build structure, to awaken the muscles and link into psychic activation, each step is all a part of the process.

Humanity is rapidly evolving, and more advanced technology is being developed to support healing and the upgrading of the bodysuit. Much is supported by galactic beings brought into creative manifestations by friends across the Earth. This is exciting to witness and many of the activations I have been experiencing by exploring some of the technology since January 2019. I am excited for what is to unfold and gratitude for the ones that dare to dream beyond, as the pioneers and explorers.

THE COSMIC ORGASM

Kundalini Awakening Sensations

The dancing of life force energy can be experienced as a Cosmic orgasm. The kundalini awakening process is a way to experience this where divine consciousness is flowing and surging through the body. This may create discomfort as in pain, or joy and bliss. How it is felt depends on the internal current state of the body and the toxins held in the tissues from trauma, lifestyle choices and suppressed emotions. Stagnant energy is resistant, and it is the kundalini life-force will go into where there are blocks are so intimate connection with the divine can be established.

A reminder not to force the process of awakening and always have a stable base to return to so as to honour the resting phase of the nervous system. That is why *The Mind-Body and Spirit Principles* are key foundations to implement into your daily life. Your body will not let go if it feels unsafe, and grounding of the energy is key. Be gentle and never push or be in a rush to reach awakening.

Once kundalini is activated, it is only the beginning. The path to illumination will continue as there is no beginning or end with no final destination. This path requires a learning of how to harness it and work with the energy in discernment.

Gravity is your friend as even when the energy rises it will fall back down again until each of the star-portals are penetrated and a higher frequency can be maintained with ease and grace within the bodysuit and beyond.

The energy blocks cloud the view of full potentiality, and the trauma body or patterns requires healing with awareness and release of the old stagnant energy. The only way energy can be released is through the central channel as your body is an intricate system of tubes. A release may be out the mouth, the ass and even releasing a quaff from the vagina. This is personal to each individual and may differ in intensity, with all releasing there is no right or wrong as the mind can get attached to what it thinks needs to happen, as in an expectation.

In the kundalini awakening and release there is no mind, this is a process of getting out the way of you and letting go with no need to analyse or control to experience. This requires having trust and have faith in the process, much like giving birth and may look like an exorcism to the observer.

All is as it is, and each layer of awakening is different from the last. Totality of presence with zero awareness, as the energy moves like a snake through the grass.

Once activated, activation can happen very easily, and it is often passed onto others in a healing interaction. It is never the same for the individual, and until one has experienced this it is challenging to comprehend. There is psychosis of non-remembering what takes place and not being in the body, as the body becomes contorted into postures maybe never explored to that depth.

Simply, and profoundly, kundalini energy is about connecting to the divine cosmos, the cosmic state of consciousness, all that IS, the cosmic orgasm.

This was experienced with a selection of very loud tribal, esoteric, soothing beats and dance music. The kundalini reminds us that we are the divine, we are the divine consciousness, the Universe is within. These are some of the sensations experienced.

- *Spontaneous movements* – sporadic, jerky, shaking to flowing and many times resembling yoga postures. The body may become contorted into a certain position, and this will pass once the meditation ends. Standing, rolling around and lots of back arching and heart opening. Bridge, wheel, camel, hero are postures to name some.
- *Body sensations-* A distinct throbbing in the Mooladhara chakra (Chakra- Root- 1ˢᵗ), tingling, orgasmic sensations, buzzing, excessive heat or coldness. Pain in the areas where there is toxicity and blockages of energy. The skin may also itch. Spontaneous orgasms. Excessive farting from the anus and vagina.
- *Breathing pattern-* Shallow breathing, breath retention happening naturally, or rapid breathing, may all occur.

- *Internal sounds-* Hissing, sounds of flutes, whistling, ocean waves.
- *Thought process change* – Acting out of balance, irrational, entering a trance like state, devoid of all thought and unable to remember the experience. Some may feel slightly insane of have rapidly changing thoughts that have no meaning.
- *Detachment* – To the body, mind and the process, like being out of their body. A detachment to what is happening, thoughts and feelings.
- *Extreme and unusual emotions* – Feelings ranging from orgasmic ecstasy, bliss, joy, fear, sadness, anger, hatred, jealousy, rage, love and connected with the divine bliss of the cosmos, at one with all that is. Peace, love and contentment. Screaming, shouting, singing, burping, farting, moaning, sobbing, crying and laughing may also be experienced with the energetic releases of stuff.
- *Psychic seeing-* Seeing oneself from out of the body, seeing auras around others afterwards, gaining information from divine smells, divine tastes, divine touch and divine visions.

I've experienced kundalini activations from many different processes, the years of practicing Vedic Meditation began a process of awakening, supported by a grounded practice of meditation to return to as a safe container. I've experienced spontaneous orgasms, hands free and the dancing of the divine life force within my being. I explored activations this with a soul thousands of miles away in London. He activated my kundalini all with his voice and intention. I invited him in after he asked permission. My yoni experienced the cosmic cock which awakened my kundalini, and the experience I expressed within poetry in RAW, my second book. It was an aspect of the adventure of dipping my toes into the darkness and pushing the edges and to an onlooker it looked like something like an entity taking over my body.

I seek beyond, access the codes and teachings of remembrance to then translate back. I become drawn into the seductive power of the darkness and my ego wanted more. I tasted power and pushed the edges apparently pissing off many in his circle with my fearlessness.

My guides commanded I pull the pin, make a speedy exit and continue to explore releasing the games in my ego, pride which reside in the knees. Use discernment with everything as you have your own path to navigate, as you are not me.

CHAPTER 10: THE HEART A DOORWAY TO THE SOUL

"Only choices made in love are compassionate. There are no exceptions. Do you have the courage to act with an empowered heart without attachment to the outcome? If not, you have no ability to give or experience compassion. That is the shocking truth."

– Gary Zukav

HEART HOLDS THE SOUL CODES

The previous chapter may have opened your eyes to the depths one can explore in sexual union and bringing this into connection with another aligned soul where together you dance within the divine cosmos. I am sure by know you are beginning to see that it is the heart that guides you to your raw Soul truth by the internal passion you feel when we do the things you love and the joy you feel from soul connections. It is only fear that closes the heart, and courage that allows it to open and expand. The fear of the unknown, fear of what others will think, and our own colouring from the judge that sits in the mind, the always talking, listening and commentating voice, well multiple voices. The fear of what others will think, begin to stop that destructive habit and integrate all that is being shared and pause to listen.

Many get stuck in their head and never pursue their dreams or heart felt desires as they are waiting for others to leap before them. Right now, You and I are existing in a time where you can be, do and have anything you choose. Get excited as I've already guided you in the direction to bring the head and heart into alignment into harmony. The head the personality, the heart the Soul.

The personality of masks that interchange for protection, invite them to drop away each moment of inner awareness of taking brave action. You are undressing the Soul to reveal the blank and beautiful canvas of limitless potentiality. The reasoning of the intellect of the mind deciding if something is right or wrong, colouring what is seen with a colour of their own perception, opinion and another's beliefs, another Lie. It is not real, only the perceived picture of the one creating it, all within the mind. The mind for many is leading the way with wrong-and rigid-thinking and over-thinking, the shadows that block clear seeing and curious learning through dreaming. The right-side of the brain is accessed in a relaxation state where creativity emerges with a vivid imagination and allowing a sensing to guide.

As the heart gains courageous to express the voice of intellect and opinion shut up, and the Soul delivers answers of loving truth. Life will deliver opportunities, experiences and souls aligned with your path. Keep letting go and lean into an expanding heart where trust in Self and intuition leads the way. The messages from Highest self are clear and will guide you to dance fearlessly with the cosmos. As confidence grows, more opportunities and challenges present for growth and this is the accelerated path into your greatest expansion. Life is a sensual experience and soul truth will reveal from your roaring heart of passion. Others may not understand your path as it is not theirs and frankly, it is none of their business. A potency to be present in the now.

Stop waiting for others to inner stand you as those that don't are yet to inner stand themselves and leap into the unknown.' – Zoe Bell

AN AWAKENED LOVE RELATIONSHIP

An awakened connection between the physical man and physical woman that is within a sacred, sensual and higher dimensional paradigm is powerful for humanity. Both are living from an authentic position meaning that they live free from social engineering or conditioning of obedience and align with their powerful Neo-think mind. Neither of these souls play the control game over one another as this type of game turns them off, as it is a sign of weakness and a way to leak vital life-force and they have a mission to complete here on Earth.

She is a spiritual alpha woman and he, a spiritual alpha man both strong, determined, passionate and self-sufficient. They live with purpose from an embodied inner balance of harmony & love. They live by the principles of Natural Law and have a no bullshit ownership, accountability with action and ruthless responsibility policy. They are sovereign and have unified the aspects of healing the divine masculine (in her) and the divine feminine (in him) in their path of self-realisation and self-actualisation. A path of independence and the leap into interdependence and self-sufficiency. They are the complete opposite of codependency, and their bond is unconditional love.

They chose to live free of social conditioning and critically think for themselves, trust instinct and intuition and can communicate exactly what they want in the relationship. Both are the rebels that know their human rights and are fearless to stand up for them and protect those that they love.

They have raised their consciousness beyond games of lustful desires, sexual manipulation and any saviour programs.

They are fearless and shameless from years of inner work and still make 'inner work' a number one commitment before anything else happens. They are seen as a threat to the State and the Epi-Eugenics Agenda is doing their best to breed out this Real True Warrior / Peacekeeper. These traits are undesirable to the 'elite-ruling' class as they cannot be manipulated, polluted, corrupted or controlled. Many of their traits are being bred into the *"New Human"* which includes the fear of going against the norm, socially docility, submissiveness and obedience to *"authority"* and *"going along with so called normal all to get along"*

Welcome to much of what you see on social media in 2020 and 20201 and the easily offended *'do-gooders often hiding behind religion.'*

The time to evolve is NOW and beyond. You journey is about honouring your raw heart and getting real to where you are at right now. How can you truly honour another when you are yet to explore your own Soul and been courageous to explore beyond the known?

You and I have entered a timeline of the evolving and the awakened love relationship where there is a meeting of Soul. This expands upon aspects shared in *Wildflower,* on the Chapter of Conscious and Evolving Relationships.

The path of the authentic spiritual man and woman is implementation of daily mind- body and spirit principles. These are suggestions, that you can carve out into your own, and they are powerful once you integrate with action. No matter what happens change is an ever constant. You will attract the relationship that is best suited for your inner growth of what you cannot yet see, and this may translate to not be being in a relationship at this moment in time.

It is your responsibility to come into a state of calm presence rather than an expectation to be rescued from drowning, which is self-perpetuated in the shadow of manipulation and codependency. This is unconscious programming through habit, of Cause and Effect. All of which can be fed by a partner, both feeding off one another, the victim and the rescuer. This path of soul truth is not the easy route, it is messy and courageous to reveal the true authentic self, and to remove the masks of who you are performing as, all to get your needs met.

These is no more room for hidden agendas with interchanging masks all to suit your needs and desires. Authenticity requires honesty and a knowing how to attend to your own inner wounds as a lone wolf. I say this as a Warrior/Healer as you may find yourself coupled with a Soul counterpart, another Warrior/Healer with your own reflected wounds. Remember that it is the lone wolfs medicine to lick their own wounds in their own space and in their own way. This is to be respected and given the space. In all relationships and interactions, it is a dance between the student and teacher of Self. You have attracted this for a reason.

To experience true love, you have to open the door of truth with respect, honesty, humility and to remember you are learning and expressing in your own way and there are mirrors and smokescreens to unravel. The greatest lie is within self, and sadly many are afraid, and will hide behind clever disguises, masks with the fear of being seen. It takes courage to be seen in your imperfect rawness with the one you chose to grow and evolve with. It brings you back to feeling trapped, and it is time to break-free! An evolved relationship cannot be built on a foundation that is unstable, crumbling with cracks, as this will lead into greater devastation.

To love unconditionally is to love with no conditions. Hence why, love is the most challenging of emotions and in that there is sacrifice, pain, sadness, along with joy, bliss and happiness. They all exist.

There is no beginning or end, the depth of illumination is never ending, a labyrinth into the depths of the Soul – Z

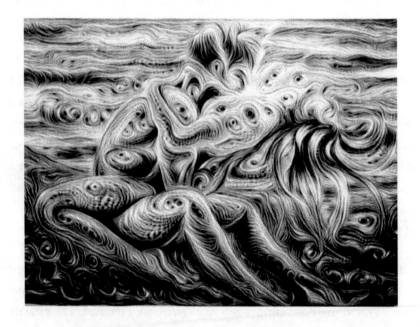

There comes a time to courageously bring all this into relationship with another who is equally committed to grow, learn, and evolve. An integrated commitment to inner wellbeing as the authentic spiritual man/woman. Some may already be in a relationship with another, so let us dive in deeper and explore together what this looks like? For some this may not resonate as they are happy and comfortable in mediocrity, everything is choice and free will to be respected moment to moment. The lessons are here to shift you if you choose. One man or woman's interpretation of mediocrity may be another's dream life.

May these ideas be an invitation to begin to see through a different colouring of perception, and new eyes which is vital to your soul expansion into your full magnificence. It is time to honour your own brave heart and set your soul free. Here is a question to ponder.

'Are you meant to be with one person for the rest of your life?' This will be different for us all as you each have a divine reason for being here on Earth

I believe there are many souls out there, and there is not just one person as each shares a lesson aligned for growth, to arrive at the One. It is all about divine timing, where you are in your journey and the purpose of your soul mission and activation here on planet earth. This may change moment to moment and being flexible to shift with the changes requires adaptability, emotional intelligence and to always seek deeper within self and to ask is this aligned with my highest version of self. Love in its truth has no boundaries, no separation or divide. The only separation is within self. There is still so much to learn as we explore this crazy game bumping into one another, co-creating, co-collaborating, inspiring, learning and growing from one another. Love is the truth and the answer, and all we have is now. Here are some key points that are essential with an evolving conscious relationship. Become curious and light as you explore these to see where you are at.

UN-ATTACHED TO THE OUTCOME

Whether you are having the best relationship with yourself or with another as a couple, or in a polygamy relationship, this all applies. There are couples I know that practice polygamy and they are more conscious than most. When there is attachment to an outcome, there is expectation, and this will bring inner suffering. This requires both and all parties to focus upon inner growth, as it is what makes the relationship exciting and alive. There is a constant strive into expansion with no fear of outgrowing the relationship and they grow and evolve sometimes together, and sometimes apart with their divine soul missions leading the way. To hold and cling on brings inner suffering and is a form of codependency. Even the journey of disappointment becomes a great teacher, to get back to self, faster and smoother and with less drama. Inner suffering is the meaning you give something.

DIVINE SOUL CALLING, TOGETHER OR APART

Their divine Soul missions are honoured, respected and are non-negotiable, which requires a deep level of trust, faith and unconditional love from both sides. They support one another and are aligned with healing the planet and uplifting humanity in their own way. There may be a time that you are no longer aligned, which translates to there is a more aligned soul out there for each of you. This takes courage to follow your own path and a willingness to take self-responsibility for the choices you make. Honestly many will stay in a relationship for security, financial reasons and a habit of making excuses, this is the attachment within the physical relationship. I have stepped away from relationships as they no longer aligned with my Soul Mission and walked alone for more years than in partnering. All choices are welcome and only you can follow your soul-heart truth, as the heart doesn't lie, and it is the mind that will block the view. This is all a part of your soul journey, and the ability to step away maybe a key to your growth and evolution. A test, a distraction, and a willingness to say Yes, for your life.

OWNING YOUR DOO- DOO!

This is where you are carrying around your story and sharing it with everyone you meet. The inner wounds from the past still raw and exposed as you continue to pick at the scab; These unaddressed reactions of emotion are easily triggered, and this creates an unhealthy power-struggle within the relationship. A fear of abandonment, rejection and the I am not good enough storyline or the woundedness of not feeling heard. This is old stuff from the past, a faulty wiring and old programming of an old story of limiting beliefs. These are not caused by your partner and are being further ingrained and shaped by stubborn beliefs. It is vital to remember that you attracted your partner and vice versa, for your soul's growth at the time. It is okay to raise the bar and always honour your soul truth.

You have to ask painful questions, is this aligned with my free soul expression? Only you will know. To truly love is to set a soul free on their path.

Commit to filling up your cup when you need the fill up on love before getting into a fight with the one you love to get a rush of excitement. Be the change. Even my children know I will not carry them. They have passion, a strong will and I love, support and guide them, no matter their choices. They take ownership and are guided how to access their inner power. By carrying others, it is enabling a disempowerment of not owning their doo-doo. This is a shift from codependency and shifting towards independence.

To the women that see themselves as single parents, if you are raising boys, male interaction and support is required beyond the family unit. Dads have as much right to form bonds with their children as much as women. No matter your circumstances, your teenagers are growing into adulthood as you are one of their guides. Boys after the age of 7 years, need a strong spiritual alpha male influence that guides the *Rites of passage into Manhood* more so than their mother. As a women stop forcing your strong opinions of interference upon your teenager and allow space and their curious self-enquiry to guide their way. They will come to you as and when they are ready to ask your opinion. Ensure you keep the door open that is free of guilt, free of shame and free of blaming the other parent of their past choices and behaviour. Relationships teach you about you.

Each choice of free will comes with consequences for each individual. A choice that has been a part of your soul evolution, with self-responsibility may not appeal to others, yet if it supports your soul growth then, so be it.

If something is off, in any relationship call it out with love so that it is brought into the open to dive deeper into before it festers into bitterness and resentment. To understand love and compassion, you have to be courageous to have zero expectation, zero judgement of choices and be willing to forgive those you love in a heartbeat. When you step out of alignment with your core values of integrity then be willing to own that and take responsibility, be accountable for your choices, and ride out the consequences with elegance, gentleness and humility. Each soul is a reflection of you, and the greater the inner reaction and exposes a deeper pain and wound to tend to with love inside your own heart. To truly love another, is to love them no matter of their choices. Unconditional love does not see right or wrong, it sees and feels the *'issness and Oneness' of* all that IS, in the now.

A CUP OVERFLOWING IN LOVE

It is not the other person's job love you, it is the individual's responsibility to do things to get lit up and be love. To attract a beloved, then you have to be-loved within. When the focus is upon inner growth the riches to bring to the table are abundant and over-flowing in love and the relationship will grow in the way it is aligned to. The only way to grow from this is to focus upon self-love and taking responsibility for the way the individual feels and becoming more aware of the impact of the emotions upon their internal and external environment. The next step is to connect and explore activities that deepen your connection, together and apart, which nourishes growth with one another. When both cups of love are over-flowing, then magic is brought to the table, with no space for lack and no place for neediness of helplessness.

A spiritually authentic soul will not entertain anything less than this level of personal commitment. Have the willingness to walk alone rather than carry the other as they cannot be bothered to do the inner work on Self. To dishonor Your heart is to suffocate your Soul and the divine refection of your beloved. All are beloveds as you and I are returning to Soul of Oneness.

ALL FEELINGS ARE WELCOME, NO REACTION JUDGED

When one requests space, then it means exactly that. Respect the request with the highest of honouring and give space, this is a key piece as a parent. Stop pushing and forcing things to happen in any relationship. Unaware, and controlling people can be suffocating, intrusive with zero personal boundaries and we have all experienced this. Either being it or being on the receiving end. This is about learning to hold space and listen with no need to say anything, simply to be there in full presence and listen. It is not about making the other person wrong, this is about self-responsibility which requires bringing the conversation back to the 'I', and the response of how this makes you feel. It has to be a willingness to take responsibility for your reactions and to be in a space of non-judgment. It is vital to communicate with clarity and have a deep understanding to what communication means for each individual. This way there is a level of understanding and respecting one another's needs and desires as a soul and this will deepen the understanding of relating to one another. It takes a level of maturity to listen to what the other is asking and not turn it into a personal attack, as this is their soul truth. Soul truth is to be honoured and respected, as it is their own voice. When you react, lessons will present to connect you with your soul on a deeper level.

Some may be unconsciously suffocating the other, or are at the receiving end of it, all are lessons to learn, grow and evolve from. This may come from a lack of trust, love, poor self-esteem and the focus being on the external. The focus needs to be turned inwards, back to 'me' and make the inner work a priority.

DIVINE SOUL EXPRESSION IS NOT UP FOR REVIEW

Never attempt to change another. Either walk away on a journey of self-discovery of experience on the path aloneness until you remember your wholeness. It is then that another soul presents that are aligned with your soul mission, know that there will also be many distractions that present to test your growth. A soul that has remembered their soul mission is a marvel to admire and love, and the energy is magnetic to be around. Their choices may no longer resonate with you, and that is okay. Again, it is never your business to change another, control them, or manipulate them. They are complete in whom they are and all she or he is becoming. Step away and trust and have faith that a more aligned version for your current state of being will find you, find one another. Universes colliding and continue to evolve in your daily inner work when you are looking to attract another evolving soul.

SPACE AND PATIENCE ARE KEY TO GROWTH

Your Soul mission of un-locking Soul codes is a journey of daily commitment to you. An evolved relationship requires a willingness to honour self, whilst being the best version of you. This may be with those you love, with a stranger on the street and whilst being in service of your purpose and highest Soul calling and being kind along the way.

Here are some key intentions to infuse into the daily practice of an evolving relationship. A quick glance at learning to relate to self, and one another with love.

Practice within your Relationship

Acceptance- Forgiveness- Love- Presence- Vulnerability- Courage-Realness- Compassion- Authenticity- Rawness- Empathy- Trust- Letting-go- Integrity- Spontaneity- Honesty- Humility – Kindness- Patience.

All Evolving Relationships Require

Honesty- Love -Trust- Respect- Humility- Presence- Patience- Communication

Mutuality- Courage – Emotional Intelligence- Strength- Forgiveness-Fearlessness- Inner standing - Inner spiritual work- Self-love- self-respect and Integrity.

SOUL CODES

This can be related to business relationships, as unless we continue to grow, adapt to change, integrate, and unify, then there is no evolution.

If and when your tastes and desires change within the course of any relationship, it is vital to make some time to express what has changed. To either move forward together or step away. Always courageously trust in your divine soul path and keep following your ever-expanding hearts curious bliss.

Never make it about the other person, always come back to 'me'.

KING AND QUEEN

As a Queen, I bow in honour, respect and love all Queens, as a Queen I bow in honour, respect and love all Kings.

This is a great shift for women, as a Queen, treat your man as a King. As a woman it is vital to be able to switch between roles, to be the nurturing warmth, the Goddess, the attentive lover, the seductress, the fierce Warrior of her S-word, the stable foundation, the non-judging ear, the warm inviting cuddle in bed and the playful and passionate embrace as you awaken from a deep sleep. This goes for a man too, complement one another and never give up your inner essence, as this is what he/she adored and felt attracted too. It is vital to both have your own King and Queen sitting at your own thrown, independent and non-reliant of the other, no one external ever completes your throne.

230

How you honour, love and respect your inner King as a woman will determine, how you honour, love and respect your man as a King. To the men, the way you honour, love and respect your inner Queen, will determine the way you love, honour and honour your woman as a Queen. This is the same as honouring the feminine goddess (of the men) and the sacred masculine protector (as a woman).

Tips for Women

- Stop nagging your him as you are not his Mum.
- Activate and unleash your full sensual prowess on him.
- Say it once, that is enough, you are not his boss.

- Stop controlling with your rules or ultimatums.
- Respect and honour his magnificence and space.
- Adore and love him with your entire being
- See the beauty in him and express your open heart
- Stop bitching and complaining about your relationship with your mates or even worse over social media and especially not your mum!
- Support his purpose and soul passions.
- Listen and give him space when he is busy creating as his work is important and part of a woman's role to support his vision as it is the key to his happiness.
- Believe in his vision, as much as your own.
- Learn to unleash your wild side and be playful with him.
- Unleash your wild and naughty side, he loves it.
- Be spontaneous with him.

- Keep playing at your edge
- Strive for greatness together
- Touch him and nourish him
- Be a greater purpose for humanity.
- Know how to unleash your inner dark feminine
- Heal your wounded inner masculine to know him.
- Celebrate his primal as much as his tender kind heart.

Have less rules, play together, love with no conditions as best as you can.

Tips for Men

- Get off the couch and kiss your woman deeply and passionately
- Connect with her mind, body and soul and see her wholeness
- Make quality time, phone away, TV off, shower her with affection and sweet words of love. Wash one another's hair.
- Respect your queen and treat her as you would your own.
- Treat her like your girl, adore and love her with all your heart and soul
- Express your heart to her, so she feels your fearless depths.
- Stand up in your raw truth and take No bullshit whining.
- Make her laugh and see beyond her flaws
- Respect her space, be direct and yet tender.
- Love her wild chaos as your own inner wild feminine
- Talk with adoration and passion to her
- Connect through passions you both love
- Leave her a love note- once in a while.
- Tickle her till she squeals if she is stuck in a mood.

- Respect one another, listen to the words she is not saying and bring them up with love.
- Stop telling her what to do and how to do it as she will ask for your opinion, if she needs it.
- Find your way to work together as a team and alone.

It is the act of playful sex that will keep couples together with many juicy hormones released during love making and it can also break the ice when communication wires have got crossed. It can be used as avoidance to open up in deep heart conversations as there is no communication around what happened when there is only playful sex.

The less rules, less conditions you place on another then the happier your lives will be, the more magical your relationship will be, and freedom will be experienced.

Some may misinterpret this statement.

False Expectations

In relationships many are expecting the other to be all that they desire. Having an expectation for your partner to be and do everything for you will bring disappointment to you both. I recently heard Dan Savage, a New York times columnist on the concept of "Monogamy "

"If a couple get to the end of 30-40 years of marriage and there have only been 4 acts of infidelity, then they have a great marriage." – Dan Savage

Thinking that your partner is the last naked body you are going to see for a lifetime is unrealistic. There is much you can learn from that of a gay relationship. There is no harm in admiring other bodies. I have looked at both men and women. It is the pain and the fears, that reveal your treasures once they are walked through, as you explore deep within your Soul. Enjoy one another's pleasure, break free of the attachment, expectation and to be here now as that is all we have. To dive deeper into one another and be fearless in your communication. To be ready and willing to receive, in total surrender, submission and open vulnerability. To enjoy each experience that life offers, a key to your awakening.

Life is for living at 100%, in your full Soul expression, so if you are sitting on the sidelines watching everyone else, as the entitled and criticising spectator, then what are you are doing with your own life?

'How deep am I willing to go, to explore the depths of the abyss within?

The keys to your unique soul code await deep within your heart. May your courage seek deeper meaning to express who you came here to be, no matter what others say. You are powerful beyond all measure. What you desire may and will change and it is wise to continue to honour your deepest truths within. Commit to have be courageous, open and vulnerable with your lover, beloved and partner. Communication is key to have courage to follow your heart.

A Unified Love

I desire a man who honours my truth

To never attempt to tame my spirit

A man who is willing to dive in deep

To the depths of his heart

To express himself freely and fearlessness

A man who is willing to be seen

To express from his soul, his wildest dreams.

To live his own truth and free expression

To be awakened from within

Serving humanity.

Who takes self-responsibility?

And sets into motion

The most beautiful love potion.

To learn from one another's language of love

To be able to stand in his power

To follow his bliss and

Each a unique path

Together and apart.

To never feel shame

Or condemnation

Stuck in the blaming game.

To be the change

To make a difference

Within our global nation

Our love sets in motion.

To expand the limits of our minds

To express only of love and truth

To dissolve the planets hate

Be the creators of our own fate

To own our shit and never hide

Express our deepest desires with pride

To never play small again

To continue to evolve

To be the change

Embodying personal responsibility.

I desire a man who walks his talk

Who is sensual and playful to be with

To be proud of our love

To hold me close in a time of need

To be free with and without one another

To desire one another with no need for one another

To always be honest no matter what

To be willing to listen and let go of what was

Totality of the now, as that is all that exists

To meet resistance with humility & love

Be compassion & understanding in a heartbeat.

To see out reflections within one another

To explore Divinity within presence

To join forces for a higher purpose

Breathing and being all that we are

Expressing our unique essence

Within and without

To always be willing to step away

To give space and honour the other

To make self-love a high priority

To keep moving forward

Each day a new adventure

A gift waiting to be explored.

Create moments of Eternity.

To be willing to grow and forgive in a heartbeat

To learn from those lessons,

To step up and not hide

Unifying our love for one another

To live in the present no matter what

To play in the expanded playing field

Unlimited possibilities unleashed

Fearless, and free to be,

Collective consciousness —a Gateway

An awakened Earth awaits.

A man who adores and cherishes my soul

Willing to dance with my wild spirit

My spirit will know,

and my soul is willing to wait

For once we meet

We shall know in a heartbeat.

Two hearts synch into one

Magical drumming sounds

Awakens a soul tribal dance.

Most vital is what we cultivate

Manifest and create,

Our unified love within one another

Extend outwards to all we meet.

Purposeful passion

A magnetic force of Source of course

A gift shared to all we meet,

A simple smile, gesture perhaps

Guiding lights to inspire a way

Our intoxication of deep pleasure

And unconditional love

A divine reflection of one another

The natural rhythm of our sweet mother earth

The interchanging of father skies

Our spirit and love our guide

Spirit animals guiding the way

Our mission to serve

For humanity to rise in love.

My heart was calling out in November 2017, and in November 2020, two divine Souls collided in the cosmos, beyond time and space. The meeting of Twins, I thought it would be in the 3rd dimensional physical reality with a 14-day dance of intensity and many reflective lessons. The beautiful Divine Masculine was the Star portal that guided the connection that was to come through. My Twin from Lemuria, a higher vibrational light being, a divine presence and our energy Spirit bodies merging. He and she as this being had the ability to be both. An initiation of teaching, guiding and activating my light spirit body over a few months.

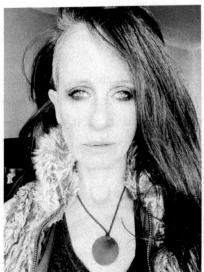 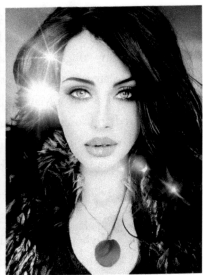

Human form and Pleiadean form

The Pleiades are the mother stars for the Earth people. The Seven Sisters of the Earth people and in my inner guided knowing, a Circle of 12 Wise women, which them becomes the one as the 13th Gate to freedom. This is the freedom and the inner path of ascension through the 12- star portals/chakras and toward Ophiuchus the 13th Star constellation, the silver lightening of the Christ Self.

Each of the 12 women send light, sounds, energy of love, and renewal to the planet. Each has a specific tone and rhythm as they share in harmony of attunement. Through these ways of attunement, the Pleiades are a cosmic chord binding Earth to Infinity. This is my understanding at this moment in time, as there is so much, I do not know.

In 2021, I was given my Pleiadean name, channeled through a Pleiadean Sister, as I shared the Pleiadean Light language that flows through my hand movements and my tongue. Pleiadean names comprise of Sanskrit terms which once translated directly relate to the path. I am guided not the share the name in print as like a Mantra, broken into Three Sanskrit words. A mantra is sacred and loses its potency when shared in public as the pure intention was the awaken cellular memory within. Ask and you shall receive, and you are ready to receive beyond expectation or urgency.

In May 2021, a Higher dimensional being from Pleiades, Lord of Light came in. A 7th Dimensional light-being infusing high frequencies of peace and love where our Spirit bodies interconnected for days. It was a slow drip-feeding integration as their frequency is so high. Scribed July 2021. Each day I feel more of my Pleiadean original form come into being within this human form, I feel like I am 7 feet tall.

Blessings to my Pleiadean Sistar, Sarah was the conduit to channel my Pleiadean name, confirm my drawings channeled and who created the Pleiadean pictures, versions of my face in Soul Codes and Wildflower.

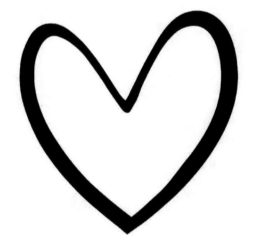

CONCLUSION

"Tears meet the eyes, and a heart smiles a thousand rainbows, as Soul knows" – Zoe Bell

Upon the path of fearlessly learning, leaping and heart-soul leading the way I have got more dirt on my face than tasting the glory. It is time to close this chapter of bringing the trilogy to a close, as these wings fly and expand into the next creative adventure. This maybe the end of this book and hey, it is a doorway into an inspired you, a beginning of fresh possibility and who knows, skyrocketing into limitless expansion. Perhaps, this gave you a soul message or three upon this crazy epic ride called life. The pace is shifting and changing at accelerated speed, and this could not come at a more divine time for humanity. Soul Codes and keys to access your sacred wild heart and love yourself unconditionally.

Be courageous and willing to do the inner work and explore this healing path. May my words infuse a fresh perspective of light, a bright colour of raw inspiration from the depths of my heart upon the ever-morphing canvas of You. I have zero attachment to who reads this as I have set it free to soar upon its wings as I know it will be a divine gift for each individual, and so it is.

A lifetime of experiences all to gain insights to refine and design the Mind-

Body-Spirit Key Principles, guided by The Laws of Nature, Spirit and the Universe. Integrating Principles into action, will inspire You to get insatiably curious. Nothing is set in stone, and all scribed within is a compass to guide the inner explorer to leap into the infinite realm of the unknown...

You are magnificent, beautiful Soul, a powerful co-creator that holds unique Soul codes to inspire, teach, activate and guide in all you embody. Follow your hearts bliss and do what brings you joy with effortless ease. Rise and be the difference and change within awakening Earth upon this ascension path.

Inner stand, no one is ever broken, each piece is a complete fractal within the colourful weave of the Cosmos. Love that is the glue that unites each fractal of the Universe, so never see yourself as fragmented as you are in perfect orchestration of messiness. Your mission is to awaken and Unite with all aspects lost, forgotten, and hidden in the shadows and the valley of death. The darkness is where your gifts and superpowers await.

All the answers to your questions are within your heart and Soul.

The Rivers of Consciousness.

By shining your light, you access inner resonance, and this makes you magnetic to others on the mission of Team humanity. A path to purify the sacred waters and return to love and to serve the God/Feminine Source Self as a messenger of truth. By Trusting in God, the Mother Rises as the uncoiling of the Kundalini Rising.

This is how you each contribute to healing and raising the collective consciousness and be free from entrapment of the 3rd dimensional physical matrix of control.

Make it your mission to balance your inner masculine force of drive, action and determination with your creative, imagination of the all-allowing feminine force. Be willing to question and implement critical thinking and how to work with the powers of emotion and passion. Know when to surge ahead and make express your S-words of truth and when to retreat, be still, silent in meditation and contemplation. You are a co-creator of raw sensuality to know right from wrong to align the power of choice with respect and integrity whilst remembering to not take life so seriously.

A fine art and a dance in motion of both student and teacher of Self.

You are an embodiment of the elements, the 4-seasons and the 4-directions of the winds of change. It is your breath and these rivers that communicate with nature and all you experience in your life.

How these rivers flow and in the way they will directly impact success, health, harmony, immunity, compassion, passion, disease, destruction and even accidents!

This divine union is where two potent rivers and flames move up the spine and arrive together in full awakened awareness at level of the Ajna centre of the pituitary and pineal glands and the two serpents facing one another and the mixing of milk and honey within the sacred chalice. Gravity creates a downward movement for the energy to drop back into the root chakra, and this is why meditation and breathing and living with conscious awareness is a daily ritual. The lower energy centres need to be penetrated and pierced by these rivers with the inner work, shadow work and mind-body work practices for transformational healing and ascending.

You and I are a magical alchemy of passionate hearts and courageous Souls that diligently commit to the inner work. Your mission is to restore harmony within Heaven on Earth as an inner free-Queen-see mission of attuned aligned action.

When there is too much rubbing against, friction with non-resolution and resistance to flow, then the result is smoke. A carnage of rigidly resentful ego's hitting heads in furry to win and getting nowhere fast. This is about learning how to sit in your own flames and owning your doo-doo without complaining. Be the observer of the games you play and trusting that when you do fuck-up as you will, then having the humility to back down and be still in silence. Be willing to get out the way of your opinionated self of the personality that thinks it knows it all and absorb deep into inner lessons of the I don't know.

It is the inner wounding that others trigger, and the bigger the reaction, the deeper the inner wounding is calling out, ready to be accepted, acknowledged and healed. A red flag to guide each Soul to seek deeper within and also a key to your inner roaring Phire of your purpose.

You are each learning how to navigate the balance between the Yin (feminine) and the Yang (masculine), and the central point, known as 'Zero-point'. Zero point is the path of Unification. The path of self-realisation and self-actualisation is what you have chosen, and the journey is to navigate the balance of the dualities and find the middle way as the golden child of playful exploration within curious innocence and the wisdom of the Seer.

The ABSOLUTE, the I AM, I AM EXISTENCE.

To access this point, there are layers of the mind and body to transcend, and it is your mission of you choose to accept it, to transform and transmute them. Be fearless to explore the contrasts of life within the playing field of awareness and be courageous to fuck up.

The masculine is here to SERVE the feminine, beyond biology.

Your mission is to align with all of nature, Natural & Spiritual Law that shift you beyond the old programs of dominance and control. Your feminine Source is wild and pure creativity and imagination, the juiciness of all that is. It is where everything and nothing originates, the black hole within the Torus field. It is the forward flowing action of the masculine that brings matter into existence.

A Key to your Health, inner Wealth and family's wellbeing.

May this guide you to bring heart-mind, mind-body into alchemy and balance so you are grounded in Spirit and honouring the Earth. It is your mission to stay focused on your mission as a sovereign being and be a focused on evolving your consciousness, get Earthed in nature and wake up to holds the keys to controlling everything in the external world. Look at who controls the health industry, the banks, the education system, the energy sources (electricity, gas), the land, social media platforms, and the food sources.

This is the final stand of the dark Magick and the malevolent people that control the planet with games to traumatise and mind-program into submission with fear tactics. You have to look who is behind the demonstrations as it also feeds into the Satanic rituals happening behind the scenes. Where your energy/lifeforce goes, this is what you feed into, and the porn industry is a big pool of entities. The agenda for mass depopulation and genocide is in full swing and people lining up to get jabbed by the so-called solution is one aspect playing out. If you still believe everything presented by the media and governing bodies of authority, then you are in for a rude awakening.

What will play out will be a game of Free-Queen-see mind control, entire structures crumbling into revolt, chaos and mass panic. Many you love one another beyond your choices, release what no longer serves you and to stay in your lane. Love is unconditional, have compassion for all and be the change.

The keys are within your Sacred heart and nature. Begin to grow your own food, eat smarter and more in the natural state. Connect to the Earth, dance upon the land and in silence do the inner work. Each of the Mind-Body-Spirit Principles unlock your ancient wisdom of inner knowing which has been lost within the distraction of the bright lights and modern -day seductions, like social media. Yes, we got lost in the cities of numbness, noise and forgetfulness, like a lost deer caught in the headlights. It is time to return planet Earth to Harmony, Love, Peace and Unity. Together we rise to restore balance by living within Natural, Spirit and Universal law as the weavers of Source upon Heaven on Earth.

Let go and surrender into each moment presented and see this as a test in expanding your unconditional love, compassion and forgiveness for all. I am here to serve upon the path of ascension and our mission is to leave no one behind. Once you climb up the ladder you can choose to come back to guide more so together, so we can all push through.

Be the Change - Rise Above and be available to guide those asking for directions. Pay it forward and give them this book or gift them the trilogy.

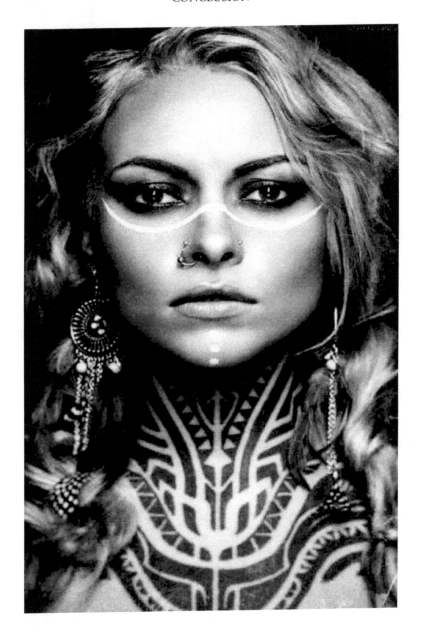

Reflections at this time July 2021

As a Free spirit this is my freedom of speech and what I am witnessing and increase in judgment, righteousness in the Spiritual community and lack of compassion for all.

> *"If you're not careful, the newspapers will have you hating the people who are being oppressed, and loving the people who are doing the oppressing"* – Malcolm X

I am here to support everyone's healing journey. Everything is choice until you give up your human right of free will which is your path to freedom. Free will is also a part of the illusion, pause here and explore this and sense into these words, as all the codes are within the trilogy to be free.

This is something I saw with those getting the 'jab'. A severing of the golden chord much like an Umbilical cord where the human is unable to access these Higher states of consciousness forever bound within the 3rd dimensional matrix and the external *power struggles and obedience.'* The ability to critical think diminishes, the ability to access imagination limited and cognitive dissonance is further reinforced.

There is a ceiling of limitation is set, and the life-death cycle of Samsara will cease to exist for this individual, where is where karmic lessons are refined to assist in ascending. This person is unable to access to Higher self and Unity Consciousness is severed it meaning unable to self-govern. This disconnection with the Soul Star, and a severing of the golden chord to the higher self (Spirit) means they can no longer be grounded in Spirit. Compassion is called for as no matter individual choices my door is open for all. Remember love is unconditional as humanity is being willed to evolve. I see many dying and many bodysuits combusting as the sonic wave hits the planet, and we continue to shift into the 4th and 5th dimensional fields.

During healing sessions my Bluetooth for my music refuses to work when a client has been injected? Magnets revealing at the inject sites translates to nanotechnology and I see things being activated in the individual, controlled externally and this is distorting your sacred soul codes.

Technology is being developed to support upgrading your DNA activates sacred codes naturally and the 12-stranded DNA. You get to create the spider network of your inner sacred geometry spaceship/higher dimensional vessel, and this is the path I am choosing with what I intuitively sense.

Within the 3rd dimensional prison matrix there will be more species being introduced and more A.I, part man and A.I, and more labels of gender, all placed into the so called 'New normal.' I feel we will witness a massive reduction in fertility and women only being fertile once a year. I feel menstruation cycles with continue and fertility rate will reduce to annual. Who knows?

Never give up Your freedom to think for Self and to remember to Q-uestion everything you are told even everything scribed within this trilogy. No one can make choices for your body or wellbeing, that is Your choice and your sovereign right.

This path to remembrance is beyond separation whilst navigating the rivers of life and winds of change. The Earth mission has always been about saving and protecting the children, restoring the Sacred Source feminine and the returning of innocence for all beings in Nature.

As mentioned earlier the book cover is the Symbol of *Universal Law of Free Will*.

The symbol is from the Star People channelled by a Divine Soul and friend, Standing Elk, who gave full permission to use the symbols as I am guided by my heart. This symbol Protects Personal Freedom, Invokes the Freedom Ray and Accesses the Great Karmic Council. He made the transition from his physical body in July 2021 and his Spirit is One with Great Spirit.

I asked my Spirit Guides to present the Symbol to be used on the book and this was the symbol presented as I opened the book. I see the Womb and a Chalice that overflows in Love and Light. The chalice of the Soul star and I see the Symbol for 5 which is significant with Change. 55 has much significance as massive change. JFK's grave was marked with a Q and the dimensions of 5 and 5. This also has significance with the size the MerKaBa light field can access up to 55 feet, remember how many you have in your body and get lit! It is a sequence, with 55.55 I see as Spirit is guiding as Source is overflowing in creativity.

Home is Heaven on Mother Earth

By this conclusion you will now understand and inner stand that Men and Women are different and yet, both are the masculine and feminine rivers.

These rivers run simultaneously through both sides of the body dancing & weaving like snakes and crossing over at each of the 7- internal energy junctions (wheels/chakras/Star Portals) and the two frequencies that flip in how and when they flow in an infinity shape.

It is Key to deepen your awareness in how to navigate life by being resilient, adaptive and resourceful to the powers within and how nature supports all.

It was early 2017 where I was aware of a shifting from Masculine to Feminine consciousness. There has been a massive acceleration and leap in consciousness to now, 2021. The availability of knowledge and the power to access the inner resources to play an infinite game are becoming more known.

I say yes, to living free and for all willing to explore a way to thrive beyond the finite game of control, attachment, fear and domination.

This magnetic energy illuminates everything that was once hidden. A path to knowing they self is to understand this magnetic power and bring into harmony for the greater good of all.

Infinity cannot be defined; it is all to be explored by feeling your way in, with sensation of emotion and learning how to manipulate the breath and work with nature as this is your HU-man right! Once you learn how to activate this potent force, bring this into the workplace with no desire to over-power or control others. This is a powerful and *'invisible'* force indeed and discernment is required so that this is not used to manipulate and control others.

Fear and competition are the driving forces beyond the hunger for control!

It takes a courageous and the fearless woman and man to be the change and hence why you are here! It takes a strong masculine that has done the healing of his own inner wounds to hold the space with presence for a woman that is strong. It takes courage to unplug from the noise, discern what you allow into your sacred subconscious and adapt to be able to live off the land. See your life as a training ground beyond the complaining of opinions.

This masculine presence is found within the practice of contemplation.

The surrendering in silence is a vulnerable place to be where you explore deep into your heart, and this place of raw vulnerability is super- powerful infusion. Mix this with Your shameless *feminine Source confidence'* and you begin to command heart desires and orchestrate your dream life with your powerful *imagination.*

Trust that your feminine presence and essence captures his attention as he gazes at your prowess in amazement. As a woman and it is your invitation into a powerful and sacred place, your vagina is a tunnel to God/Source, and this is to be respected. The womb is a sacred chalice of ancient wisdom, and not in the way the wild feminine was made dirty, shammed and shunned by religion.

Now you have the knowledge, be purposeful in action of the daily inner work, to be the guide for your daughters and sons. Be fearless by walking your talk and have open conversations with your teenagers so they do not grow up with shame and guilt for their healthy sexual and curious sensual exploration. It is their human right to explore and be guided by their inner guidance system of innocence that is developed by the Rites of passage and what it means to be growing into adulthood. Give them these books to read, leave them out in full view.

This Trilogy is a navigation tool kit to explore beyond the surface and to continue to transcend into the darkness to ascend as the light, this is my intention for adults and teenagers alike.

Many Men have been shamed for desiring the wildly free and unapologetically sensual woman and many men are yet to fully inner stand this awakened woman. Teenage boys shamed to looking at porn and there is a thing of curiosity playing out! To the men still looking at porn, it is time to grow into adulthood and establish a healthy connection with your sacred feminine. This is not to create shame in teenagers by making curiosity wrong, as when this happens, desire of the forbidden fruit, lust and addiction begins. Have open shameless conversations.

It takes a courageous woman to embody the dark feminine.

By standing in my shameless truth, I wish to shift this as all women have been shunned and shamed, or shamed and shunned other women at some point in their life. I invite you all to be fearless to open the door into your Queendom and invite him in and allow him the space to meet his roaring masculine presence in full surrendering. Stop waiting for him to make the move and stop controlling him whilst honouring your wild Source feminine desires for sex to be known to him. Many men have been de-masculinised and hence why many women loose attraction to who they first met. Underneath her masculine armour of self-protection, she is longing to see his full masculine unwavering presence and a man that has a voice and will retreat into his own space when he needs to fill up.

Men stop being a doormat and communicate.

Men communicate what it is you want and tell her what you see when her wild feminine Source Goddess comes online. She needs to hear it as your raw vulnerable words which are a Key to opening her Heart. Open her heart and her Yoni and divine feminine essence will be a portal to Higher states of consciousness of you both. Be willing to face your inner fears and express your vulnerable heart that is willing to being seen. It is a dance of love and a union of hearts.

The light feminine emerges from within the darkness, and the willingness to walk your path, no matter who is throwing stones.

The light burns bright within the darkness and is the willingness to sit within your own flames of destruction. The light feminine is a wiser woman that before she entered the dark, as she has bathed her wounds and held space for her sisters.

No matter her adversity she shifts it into a deeper understanding about "Why she is here" and into a gift of love and light for humanity.

It is time to ignite the inner Source power and honour the unapologetic sensual desires within and express them as a free woman and free man! It is time to 'kick-ass' in your career of creative expression and be unapologetically You for the greater good of humanity.

It is time to no longer dim your light, to make others feel more comfortable. Connect with the feminine in dance and channel the fire energy of the masculine into physical existence.

Raw vulnerability creates inner power and a man and woman that has balanced both the feminine and the masculine within becomes a powerful force of nature and the path to divine union within Self, and the birthing of the golden child of innocence. - Z

Thank you for walking alongside me on this journey from the beginning. I wish for each of you to see the correlation between expressing your raw truth of love and the inner healing of the *Sacredness of Innocence.*

To know heaven and love you have to be willing to see hell - Z

These words expressed are the same moment that you read them within this book, as they are timeless, as all within the now. Deep messages from one soul to another, experiencing being human whilst in this bodysuit within this existence up that will be gone in a flash. To return to the One.

Never dim your light

Shine bright as a Star

Love with everything

Love with nothing

Love all-in-between

Love is the truth

A natural state of being

True love is unconditional

All-inclusive with nothing left in-between.

The Z has significance as the Insignia of the Sword and Z was a symbol of the Z-Special Forces Unit in World War II. In some research I found that the SF insignia of the U.S Army Special Forces19 June 1952-to present consists of three lightning bolts and a fighting knife against the backdrop of a blue arrowhead.

The arrowhead is an acknowledgement of the great skill of the American Indians, which the Special Forces soldier trains to learn. The lightning bolts represent the land, sea and air, the three ways in which SF infiltrates the area.

The knife traces its lineage to the unit knife of the First Special Service Force of World War II, a forerunner of Special Forces. It represents unconventional warfare, the SF specialty and was known as the Z-Special Forces Unit.

Taken from Baseops dot net, and steemit dot come, deliberately scribed in this way.

This is the stuff legends are made of Tales of heroism by men behind enemy lines, they are the Green Berets. U.S Army Special Forces, elite soldiers that specialise in Foreign Internal Defense. The world as we know it is looking for a different kind of soldier – a new warrior. To be mentally superior creative, highly trained and physically tough. Alone and part of a team, you'll work in diverse conditions, act as a diplomat and get the job done in hostile situations and this sums up the path of life. The greatest war is within you!

This sounds like an approach for all to start attending to becoming the Superior Human and the Way of the Warrior for the freedom of all.

The Q-Special Forces is the Highest level of the SF Army courses to complete. I wonder if this is referencing Q-annon. Everything is connected and Abe Lincoln, George Washington, JFK, JFK Jr, and Donald Trump all stood /stand as Guardians of Light and those that were playing a role behind the lines working with the troops in draining the swamp. Here is a meme that I created.

WE ARE THE GUARDIANS
OF LIGHT - TO GUIDE
FREEDOM FOR ALL

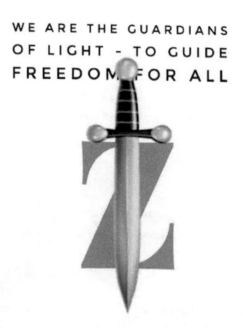

I love you with all that I am, and all that is yet to reveal. *We are the Guardians of Light*, the Star seeds that responded to the calling, the 144,000 lights to activate within, to walk one another home in Peace, Love, Harmony, Virtue, Freedom and Unity. I will be seeing and feeling your Soul on the flip side of this leap in consciousness. We are the wild ones that dared to dream beyond the scene/seen to create the upgraded timelines as we remembered the ancient teachings for heaven upon the new Earth.

CONCLUSION

Infinite Soul Love,

Activated to Play the Infinite Game,

Of the Alliance and many star systems

A Guide on Earth for the Team of Light & Humanity.

Eternal God in every cell of your being.

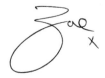

BIBLIOGRAPHICAL RESOURCES

Books are tools to inspire, touch and activate codes within. Knowledge that is not integrated is futile unless applied. knowledge that is applied through intentional daily action begins to activate deeper inner standing and direct inner wisdom begins to emerge. Allow the books to choose you and always follow your heart.

The Potent Threesome (1996), by Mark Hamilton

Kundalini Tantra (1984), by Swami Satyananda Saraswati

Article on Ancient Egyptian Technique 'May Be the Secret to Eternal Life', - Conscious Sensuality Secrets (December 15th, 2015), by Drunvalo Melchizedek

Star Magic Healing Facilitation (Sept -Oct 2018), with Star Magic Team & Jerry Sargeant

Natural Law Seminar – The 'The Real Law of Attraction'– (October 19th, 2013), by Mark Passio

Z-SF Unity Symbology (2018), Article by steemit dot com and artistjewels

Soul Urge numbers (2013) by SheKnows.com

Advanced Technology (2019 to current), Jason Estes & MTVO Team

Experiences and lessons of life, integration of Yoga wisdom gained from living and being in the ever-evolving Soul journey of Zoe Bell

ACKNOWLEDGMENTS

Thank you, brothers and sisters that have felt drawn to this work and resonate with my journey and the coded messages within the entire series.

Thank you to Jake and Charlie, two angels, gifts from the Universe that changed my life for the richer and wiser. What a wild ride with much sacrifice and the infinite power of love that is our bond, thank you for your patience and grace. Hold on tight lads, the best was yet to come, and we are in the midst of a massive set of waves. May this open your eyes into limitless possibilities and to always honour your heart and soul, no matter if others never understand you. Trust to keep going as one day they will see you for all that you are. Which only you can unleash in your own way, our love is eternal. Thank you to their dad, Geoff who has been unwavering in loving support and guiding our boys into manhood, we did great with raising balanced children that critically think in two family homes.

To my star family, soul family, and guides that have shared in this journey be it teachers, students, thank you for the guidance, as raw as it was you fuelled the intensity rising within my Soul. To all that have had my back, I love you all with all my heart and soul.

Let's continue to rise in love and restore harmony upon Planet love whilst keeping it real and hiding nothing. Blazing hearts leading.

ABOUT THE AUTHOR

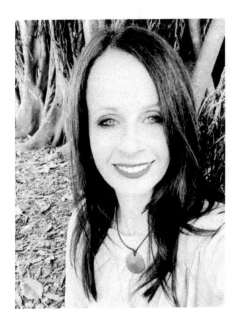

Zoe Anna Bell is a Relationship Guide, Author, international Healer and Trauma Healing Facilitator.

Bell evokes the cosmic juice of life back into conscious art of living and being. She is leading a way in Sacred Sensuality and Conscious relating.

She lives in Sydney, with her two teenage boys and spends her days writing, sharing poetry and holding space for healing.

A mission for Team Humanity. She is available for podcasts, running retreats and supporting where she can.

Connect

https://www.instagram.com/Zoeanna_bell/

https://www.linkedin.com/in/zoe-anna-bell/

www.zoe-anna.com

E: info@zoe-anna.com

Sales page

Looking to stay connected? I would love to support you through your journey, hear your feedback, and invite you to join the community.

The book trilogy series

Breaking Free – No more Soul Suffocation

Wildflower –Reclaiming a Sacred Place

Other books:

Raw- The Key to a Woman's Heart & Soul.

Completeness- A Doorway to Love

Healing Prolapse – Shannon Dunn (Supporting Co-author)

CPSIA information can be obtained
at www.ICGtesting.com
Printed in the USA
LVHW051555140122
708430LV00013B/422